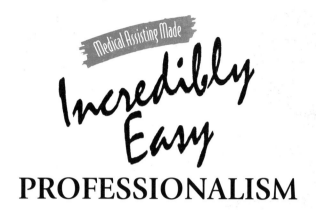

PROFESSIONALISM

D1616208

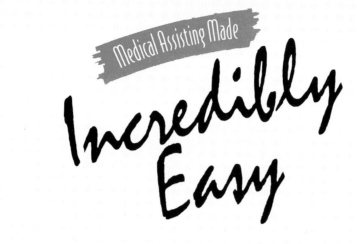

Medical Assisting Made

Incredibly Easy

PROFESSIONALISM

Jackie Marshall, MEd

Tri-State Educational Systems, Inc.
Ohio Business College
Ohio Institute of Health Careers
Lorain, Ohio

Wolters Kluwer | Lippincott Williams & Wilkins
Health
Philadelphia · Baltimore · New York · London
Buenos Aires · Hong Kong · Sydney · Tokyo

Executive Editor: John Goucher
Senior Managing Editor: Rebecca Kerins
Marketing Manager: Nancy Bradshaw
Production Editor: Eve Malakoff-Klein
Illustrator: Bot Roda
Designer: Joan Wendt
Compositor: Circle Graphics, Inc.
Printer: C&C Offset Printing

351 West Camden Street   530 Walnut Street
Baltimore, MD 21201   Philadelphia, PA 19106

Printed in China

9 8 7 6 5 4 3 2 1

Library of Congress Cataloging-in-Publication Data

Marshall, Jackie.
   Professionalism / Jackie Marshall.
      p. ; cm.—(Medical assisting made incredibly easy)
      Includes index.
      ISBN 978-0-7817-7210-5
   1. Medical assistants—Professional ethics. 2. Medical assistants—Vocational guidance. I. Title. II. Series.
      [DNLM: 1. Allied Health Personnel. 2. Professional Practice. 3. Professional-Patient Relations. W 21.5 M3678 2009]
      R728.8.M317 2009
      610.73′7069—dc22

                              2007042526

To purchase additional copies of this book, call our customer service department at **(800) 638-3030** or fax orders to **(301) 223-2320**. International customers should call **(301) 223-2300**.

Visit Lippincott Williams & Wilkins on the Internet: http://www.lww.com. Lippincott Williams & Wilkins customer service representatives are available from 8:30 am to 6:00 pm, EST.

PREFACE

Medical Assisting Made Incredibly Easy is an exciting new series designed to make learning enjoyable for medical assisting students. Each book in the series uses a light-hearted, humorous approach to presenting information. Maria, a Certified Medical Assistant, guides students through the books, offering helpful tips and insight along the way.

Medical Assisting Made Incredibly Easy takes a practical approach, providing students with the critical information that they need to know, including complete coverage of the core skills they must master in their studies. The series covers all competencies based on the standards and guidelines established for medical assisting by the Commission on Accreditation of Allied Health Educational Programs (CAAHEP) and the Accrediting Bureau of Health Education Schools (ABHES).

About This Book

Medical Assisting Made Incredibly Easy: Professionalism provides students with a solid understanding of the importance of professionalism in the classroom and the workplace, covering essential topics such as professional appearance, communication skills, customer service, cultural diversity, and job search skills. The text covers ABHES's "Professionalism" competencies, as well as a variety of CAAHEP competencies related to this topic. These are among the skills that students must master to pass the test required to become either a Certified Medical Assistant or a Registered Medical Assistant.

Special Features

Medical Assisting Made Incredibly Easy: Professionalism is designed to be enjoyable to read, as well as highly informative. Each chapter in this book includes special features designed to guide students in their study. These elements will help students identify the most important information in the chapter and to understand all of it.

 • *Road Map to Success* includes a list of skills and other important information that students will gain after reading the material.

 • *Chapter Competencies* highlights the ABHES and CAAHEP competencies covered in each chapter.

 • *Signs & Signals* includes special tips, clues, and hints from a more experienced mentor.

 • *Road Rules* summarizes key points to remember about a particular skill or trait.

 • *Ask The Professional* offers expert advice on how to handle difficult situations that medical assistants may face in the workplace.

 • *Travelog* highlights learning experiences and revelations encountered by a medical assisting student as she travels on her journey from beginning student to employed, certified medical assistant.

 • *Fork in the Road* offers students a critical thinking exercise to complete.

 • *Running Smoothly* features situations that medical assistants may encounter in a medical office and shows how students can apply what they have learned to those situations.

 • *Journey's End* summarizes a chapter's key content.

 • *Map Your Progress* tests students on what they have learned via an end-of-chapter quiz.

In addition to the above features, this book also includes bolded key terms throughout each chapter and a Glossary in the back of the book, as well as many other boxed features and tables.

Additional Resources

In addition to the text, the following resources are available for instructors:

- An **Instructor's Resource CD-ROM** with test generator, PowerPoint slides, answers to end-of-chapter quizzes, case studies, and customizable competency evaluation forms helps instructors optimize their teaching.
- A complete set of **Lesson Plans** is also available to instructors.

Medical Assisting Made Incredibly Easy: Professionalism is designed to make the study of professional conduct fun and effective. The purpose of this book, and the entire *Medical Assisting Made Incredibly Easy* series, is student success!

USER'S GUIDE

Hello, my name is Maria. I'm a Certified Medical Assistant and educator, as well as your guide through this textbook. There are a number of features in this **Medical Assisting Made Incredibly Easy** text to help you learn everything you need to become a successful medical assistant. Read through this User's Guide to orient yourself to everything the text has to offer. Good luck in your medical assisting studies!

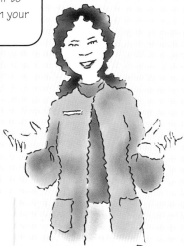

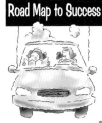

Road Map to Success

- Identify possible obstacles to employment as a medical assistant, and explain how to overcome them

- Explain how to determine your ideal medical assisting job

- Establish realistic goals for your future

- Describe basic job search methods, including how best to utilize available resources

- Create effective resumes and cover letters, and explain the benefits of these job search tools

- Explain how effective communication skills and proper interviewing techniques will assist you in getting hired as a medical assistant

- List the factors to consider when deciding whether to accept or decline a job offer

Road Map to Success orients you to the material that's covered in the current chapter.

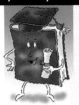

Chapter Competencies

- Be attentive, listen, and learn (ABHES 2.a.)
- Be courteous and diplomatic (ABHES 1.h.)
- Adapt what is said to the recipient's level of comprehension (ABHES 2.c.)
- Instruct individuals according to their needs (CAAHEP 3.c.3.b.)
- Be impartial and show empathy when dealing with patients (ABHES 2.b.)

Chapter Competencies tell you which skills are covered in each chapter, as outlined by CAAHEP and ABHES.

Signs & Signals

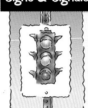

POSTING YOUR RESUME ON THE WEB

Most job search sites allow you to conduct a search for jobs in your area. You can do so by simply entering the title of the position you're seeking and any other relevant keywords into the search bar. But did you know that some sites not only allow job seekers to search advertisements; they also allow potential employers to search for qualified candidates? Right now, your next employer might be searching for a candidate like *you!*

Popular job search sites, such as CareerBuilder.com, give job seekers the option to post their resumes online. It's usually a very simple process.

1. First, click on the appropriate "Post Resume" link.
2. Next, click on "Browse" to locate your resume file on the computer. If you're using a computer in your campus library or computer laboratory, insert the disk or CD containing your resume file before clicking on "Browse."

Signs & Signals boxes include special tips, clues, and hints from a more experienced mentor.

Road Rules

CULTURAL DIVERSITY AND THE MEDICAL ASSISTANT

It's important to be sensitive to cultural diversity in the medical office. Cultural diversity is multilayered and serves several functions in a person's life. In the health care setting:

- A patient's diet and nutrition is a vital component of her health care. A patient's genetics can also predispose her to certain medical diseases or disorders.
- Everyone feels pain, but culture influences how people choose to express pain. Watch for discrepancies between how a patient says she feels and what her body language is telling you.

Road Rules boxes summarize key points to remember about a particular skill or trait.

Ask The Professional ACCOMMODATING PATIENTS

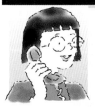

Q: *How can I accommodate patients who aren't the decision makers in their family?*

A: Patients who don't make their own health care decisions may seem reluctant to offer suggestions or information. Ask to speak with the decision maker directly, in the presence of the patient. Make sure that you explain all information thoroughly and accurately to both individuals. The patient may want to discuss the information with the decision maker in private.

Ask The Professional boxes offer expert advice on how to handle difficult situations that you may face in the workplace.

Travelog WORKING WITH A PRECEPTOR

As a medical assisting student with no experience in a medical setting, I was nervous about completing the externship. I'd never practiced my skills outside the classroom or even seen some of the equipment I would be using, except in textbooks. I felt relieved when I learned that a preceptor would be working closely with us. The preceptor was so helpful! She put me at ease by explaining procedures and techniques in detail and answering my questions. Once, during training, I was asked to take an infant's blood pressure. I was so afraid of hurting him! My preceptor showed me where to place the blood pressure cuff and how to read it. I felt much better knowing that I could ask for help if I needed it. Her assistance was similar to that of the classroom instructor, which helped make my transition from the classroom to the medical office that much smoother. My preceptor was an invaluable help to me during my externship experience!

Travelog boxes highlight learning experiences and revelations encountered by an African American medical assisting student as she travels on her journey from beginning student to employed, certified medical assistant.

Fork in the Road PROVIDING AGE-APPROPRIATE CARE

On the next page, match each age group in the first column with the medical assistant's correct behavior from the second column. Then, in one to two sentences, explain why each behavior is correct in terms of the child's stage of development.

Fork in the Road boxes challenge you with a critical thinking exercise to complete.

Running Smoothly

KEEPING IT PROFESSIONAL

What if a patient misinterprets your friendliness as flirtation?

Most patients will appreciate a friendly and cheerful attitude. But sometimes, people can mistake a friendly touch or kind gesture as something more. If you feel that a patient has misinterpreted something you've said or done, then explain what you meant. If the person persists, then firmly state that your relationship must remain professional. Remaining firmly within the legal and ethical boundaries of your position will help you provide the best possible health care to patients.

> Friendliness can sometimes be mistaken for flirtation, but don't let that keep you from reaching out when you feel a patient needs therapeutic touch.

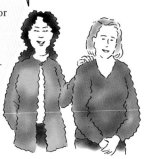

Running Smoothly boxes feature situations that you may encounter in a medical office and teach you to apply what you've learned to those situations.

Journey's End summarizes a chapter's key content.

Journey's End

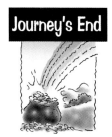

- You may be faced with obstacles to employment as a medical assistant, such as a lack of experience, gaps in your employment, or being fired from a previous job. Maintaining a positive attitude is one way to overcome these obstacles.

- Set goals for yourself by determining your ideal job. Think about the many elements that make up each job and describe the type of position you'd like to find. Consider the type of facility where you'd like to work, which duties you'd like to perform, and what your ideal working hours would be.

- Set realistic career goals for yourself by researching estimated industry growth and typical salaries for medical assistants. In terms of position and income, decide where you'd like to be in the next two to five years.

Map Your Progress

Answer the following multiple-choice questions.

1. Which of the following is *not* a good reason to provide for gaps in your employment?
   a. schooling
   b. relocation
   c. long commute
   d. pregnancy

2. Which of the following individuals would make the *best* reference?
   a. best friend
   b. rabbi

Map Your Progress provides you with a short quiz so you can test your knowledge.

REVIEWERS

Julie Akason
Argosy University
Eagan, Minnesota

Nina Beaman
Bryant and Stratton College
Richmond, Virginia

Tracie Fuqua
Wallace State Community College
Hanceville, Alabama

Christine Golden
Waukesha County Technical College
Pewaukee, Wisconsin

Carolyn Helms
Atlanta Technical College
Atlanta, Georgia

Rebecca Hickey
Butler Technology and Career Development Schools
Fairfield Township, Ohio

Joanna Holly
Midstate College
Peoria, Illinois

Dorothy Kiel
Rhodes State College
Lima, Ohio

Deeann Knox
Ivy Tech Community College
Fort Wayne, Indiana

Christine Malone
Everett Community College
Everett, Washington

Maureen Messier
Bradford Hall Career Institute
Southington, Connecticut

Lisa Nagle
Augusta Technical College
Augusta, Georgia

Linda Romines
Ivy Tech Community College
Fort Wayne, Indiana

Amy Semenchuk
Rockford Business College
Rockford, Illinois

Lynn Slack
Kaplan Career Institute
Pittsburgh, Pennsylvania

Cheryl Startzell
San Antonio College
San Antonio, Texas

Nina Thierer
Ivy Tech Community College
Fort Wayne, Indiana

Stacey Wilson
Cabarrus College of Health Sciences
Concord, North Carolina

CONTENTS

Chapter 1

THE ROAD TO PROFESSIONALISM

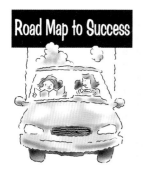

Road Map to Success

- Define professionalism

- Explain the role of professionalism in the journey to become a successful medical assistant

- List five effective study and test-taking skills that can help you get the most out of your educational experience

- Identify character traits that are important to develop as a successful medical assistant

- Summarize how self-assessment can help you identify personal changes you may need to make to become a successful medical assistant

- Explain why a responsible attitude is important in your role as a medical assistant

- Describe ways of showing initiative in the workplace

- Describe the critical thinking process

- Explain the importance of critical thinking in the medical office

- List three team-playing skills that are important to practice in your role as a medical assistant

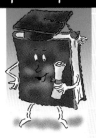

Chapter Competencies

- Identify professional components (ABHES 2.p.)
- Identify the importance of credentialing for allied health professionals (ABHES 2.q.)
- Project a positive attitude (ABHES 1.a.)
- Evidence a responsible attitude (ABHES 1.g.)
- Exhibit initiative (ABHES 1.e.)
- Maintain confidentiality at all times (ABHES 1.b.)
- Identify and respond to issues of confidentiality (CAAHEP 3.c.2.a.)
- Be a "team player" (ABHES 1.c.)

What makes a professional, and why is professionalism in the medical office so important? In this chapter, you'll learn exactly what professionalism is and how it can help you on the road to becoming a successful medical assistant. Learning how to be a professional is an important part of medical assisting.

What Is Professionalism?

Professionalism is the attitude of being a professional, that is, of having a positive outlook and a commitment to doing your best at all times. In the medical office, professionalism is the ability to use your knowledge and skills to secure the interests and welfare of the patients you care for. Make sure that you look and sound professional, as medical assisting is about the whole package. A medical assistant who demonstrates professionalism will:

- display a respectful manner and image
- dress appropriately
- demonstrate initiative and responsibility
- work effectively as a member of the health care team
- prioritize and perform multiple tasks well
- adapt to change
- enhance skills through continuing education
- treat all patients with compassion and empathy
- complete accurate and thorough work

- follow all office policies and procedures
- safeguard the confidentiality of private patient information
- promote the practice of medical assisting through positive public relations

Education and Credentialing

Education is the first step toward becoming a professional. Before you begin your career in the medical field, you'll need to acquire the knowledge, skills, and credentials that will prepare you for your journey as a medical assistant. A professional student takes her education seriously and develops the experience and know-how to face challenges head-on. Once you've acquired an education, you'll transition from student to working professional—although the learning never ends. First, let's take a look at the things you'll need to reach your goal.

You'll gain experience as a student before tackling professional challenges.

STUDENT DRIVER

TOP OF THE CLASS

Congratulations! You've decided to obtain an education that will take you where you want to go. The classes you'll take will guide you on your path to becoming a professional medical assistant, so it's important to learn all you can as a student. The more you learn now, the better prepared you'll be when handling patient concerns within a professional health care setting.

Medical Assisting Programs

The medical assisting program you've chosen may be:

- a six-month to one-year program, for which you'll receive a certificate of graduation or diploma
- a two-year program, for which you'll receive an associate's degree

Why choose a two-year program when you could obtain a diploma in only six months? The benefit of participating in a two-year program is the additional knowledge you'll gain. Programs that offer an associate's degree usually include general studies (such as English, math, and computer skills), as well as core courses specific to medical assisting (such as medical terminology and insurance coding). These programs not only help you learn the things you'll need to know as a medical assistant, they also help you gain other valuable skills. By developing good writing, math, and computer skills, you'll give yourself an advantage in the work force.

Accreditation

Many schools seek accreditation for their medical assisting programs. **Accreditation** is a process that evaluates educational programs for quality based on academic and administrative standards. It's a "seal of approval" that is granted to a school with a curriculum that meets these standards. Accredited medical assisting programs include:

- general studies, such as English, math, and computer skills, as well as core courses, such as medical terminology and insurance coding
- an **externship,** in which you'll work in a professional setting to gain hands-on experience

Accrediting Organizations

Two organizations currently accredit medical assisting programs:

- the **Commission on Accreditation of Allied Health Education Programs (CAAHEP)**
- the **Accrediting Bureau of Health Education Schools (ABHES)**

These two organizations identify specific competencies, or skills, that accredited medical assisting programs must teach students. You may already be familiar with the acronyms CAAHEP and ABHES because many of your classes are focused on the importance of mastering these competencies.

What are the benefits of attending an accredited program? One is that accreditation ensures that the school's curriculum covers the necessary information and skills you'll need to have as a professional. Another is that attending an accredited school is sometimes a requirement for certification.

CERTIFICATION

Certification is a sign of excellence. **Certification** proves that you've completed an approved program and mastered the skills you'll be expected to perform in the workplace. Professional organizations, such as the **American Association of Medical Assistants (AAMA)** and the **American Medical Technologists (AMT),** create the standards for certification.

Certification is a voluntary process, which means it's not required for you to get a job. However, an increasing number of physician's offices, are seeking out and hiring trained and certified medical assistants.

You'll learn more about certification and renewal in Chapter 7. But first, let's take a look at what it takes to become certified by the AAMA or the AMT.

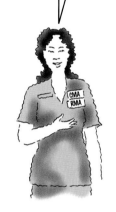

CMA and RMA credentials let potential employers know that you have a commitment to professionalism.

Becoming a Certified Medical Assistant

Medical assistants who meet the requirements established by the AAMA can become certified medical assistants (CMAs). To receive certification, you must:

- graduate from a medical assisting program that is accredited by CAAHEP or ABHES
- complete an externship as part of the medical assisting program
- pass the AAMA CMA Certification Examination

The CMA credentials are nationally recognized and don't require any action when moving from one state to another. However, you must obey the specific laws governing medical assistants in the state where you work.

Becoming a Registered Medical Assistant

Medical assistants who are certified by the AMT receive the title of registered medical assistant (RMA). To apply for certification, you must:

- be at least 18 years old and of good moral character
- hold a diploma from an accredited high school (or acceptable equivalent)
- graduate from a CAAHEP or ABHES accredited medical assisting program or possess at least five years' experience as a professional medical assistant (with no more than two years as an instructor)

Once these requirements have been met, you must then pass the AMT Certification Examination to receive certification and become an RMA.

CONTINUING EDUCATION

Once you finish your program, that doesn't mean your education has to end, too. Professional medical assistants continue their education by taking courses and seminars on various topics in the field. If you're pursuing a career as an administrative medical assistant, you might want to take courses on new computer programs or software and technology that will help you in the office. Other common topics covered in **continuing education** courses include:

- unfamiliar clinical procedures
- new laws and regulations
- pharmaceutical updates

Some employers pay for medical courses and seminars. If not, you may be able to include these costs for a tax credit when filing your annual income tax return. More details about continuing education will be discussed in Chapter 7.

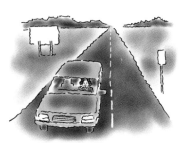

For professionals, learning is a lifelong endeavor.

DIRECTIONS FOR STUDENT SUCCESS

As a student, the path to success isn't always easy. Along the way, you'll inevitably encounter challenges. But if you're equipped with a positive attitude and the right skills, you'll be able to face these challenges head-on and stay on the path to success. To be a successful student, you'll need to develop and maintain:

- a positive attitude
- time management skills
- study skills
- test-taking skills

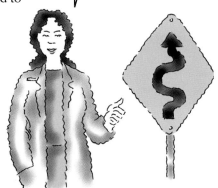

The path to success can have many twists and turns. But a positive attitude and the right skills will help you find your way!

The Right Attitude

Your **attitude** is your state of mind, how you're feeling, or your perspective. As a student, it's important to have a positive attitude so you're open to new information and ready to take on the challenges and tasks ahead of you.

Taking responsibility for your personal success and your education will help you remain dedicated to achieving your goals. Everyone has bad days now and then, but a consistently negative outlook can prevent you from reaching your potential. The following tips will help you develop and maintain a positive attitude.

- Learn to rely on a support system. Fellow students, friends, family members, and instructors can be excellent sources of support during your education.
- Get plenty of rest, proper nutrition, and exercise. Being healthy and feeling good about yourself will help you stay positive.

- Stay motivated by setting and then focusing on goals. Rewarding yourself each time you reach a new goal can give your attitude a boost.
- Think positively. Believing you can do something is the first step toward accomplishing it.

Goals

In school, it can be difficult to concentrate and stay motivated if you don't have clear goals in mind. A goal is an objective that you work hard to reach. Goals not only help you avoid distraction, but they give you something to reach for. When you can see how your daily tasks relate to your goals, you begin to understand why each task is important.

For example, during a particularly busy week, you may not feel like completing an assignment. "What's the point?" you might ask yourself. Relating the task to one of your goals—for example, earning a B in a particular course—might give you the motivation you need to complete it. By imagining how the task at hand will help you achieve a specific goal, it's easier to see how each step takes you closer to your goal of becoming a successful medical assistant. And as you accomplish your goals, you'll gain confidence and move forward on your journey to success.

Creating goals helps you map out the course to your destination: professional medical assistant.

Set Yourself Up for Success

When developing goals for yourself, include a wide variety. You may have one or two long-term career goals as well as several short-term goals that you plan to accomplish along the way. For example, suppose one of your long-term goals is to work as a medical assistant in a pediatrician's office. To accomplish that goal, you'll need to set several short-term goals for yourself. Here are three realistic short-term goals you might set for yourself:

- taking the required courses
- developing your skills in an externship
- applying for certification

Before you jump right in, make sure you're setting yourself up for success. The goals you set should be:

- *Measurable.* Is each goal specific and easily measured? Have you set tentative deadlines for accomplishing your goals? For example, "I will read ten pages for biology class before Wednesday" is a more specific goal than "I want to do well in biology class."

Road Rules — SETTING GOALS

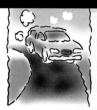

- Setting goals helps you to stay motivated and on track for success.
- Goals should be measurable, achievable, and desirable.
- Anticipate potential problems in meeting each goal, and create a plan to avoid or overcome them.
- Start by setting small goals that are simple and practical.
- Reaching smaller goals paves the way for reaching larger goals in the future!

- *Achievable.* Are your goals realistic, given your skills, strengths, and resources? Have you given yourself enough time to achieve each goal? Keep in mind that your goals can be modified and changed if necessary.

> Remember to evaluate and revise your goals as needed. Your goals are meant to serve you, not the other way around!

- *Desirable.* Do your goals represent things *you* want (instead of what *others* may want for you)? Will accomplishing each goal take you one step closer to where you want to be?

Revise Your Goals

Part of staying on the path to success includes reviewing your goals from time to time and revising them as necessary. Make sure your goals will help you move in the direction you want to go. If they aren't, change them as necessary.

If you fail to accomplish a goal, avoid becoming discouraged. Instead, take the opportunity to evaluate the goal. Ask yourself:

- Was this goal measurable, achievable, and desirable? If not, what revisions need to be made?
- Do I need to set a more realistic deadline for accomplishing this goal?
- What challenges prevented me from accomplishing this goal as planned? How can I overcome these challenges?

Reward Yourself

Above all, reward yourself for each goal you accomplish. Rewards, whether small or large, can motivate you to keep pur-

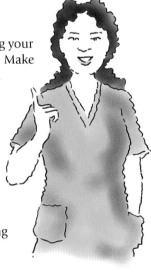

suing your goals. Just remember to choose rewards that are proportionate to the task completed.

You may find that the best reward for doing well on a school assignment is simply allowing yourself an extra half-hour of relaxation time in the evening. Or maybe the promise of a night out with friends will motivate you to study for a test. Think about what things motivate you to keep going, and then reward yourself for a job well done!

Time Management

You are likely committed to many personal and professional goals and obligations. Now you've added one more responsibility to your plate: student. How are you going to get everything done?

The following suggestions will help you manage your time wisely.

- Make a list of things you need to accomplish each day and then prioritize them. Which items on your list are the most urgent and need to be done immediately, and which can you save for later?
- Be prepared. Know what is expected of you, such as what you'll need to study, class requirements, and so forth, so that you can meet all your deadlines on time.
- Find a balance. Working too hard can cause unnecessary stress. Remember to take some time out for yourself.
- Seek out support. Let your family and friends know about your other time commitments, and ask for help when you need it.

Map Your Schedule

Successful students know the importance of having good work habits, such as planning and organizational skills. When you plan and organize your time commitments, you are scheduling. Schedules are like maps: they can show you how far you've come and how much further you need to go to reach your goals.

Scheduling frees you from the anxiety that comes with feeling unprepared. An effective schedule can help you plan when to do something and how much time to budget for the task, as well as identify other tasks that you need to accomplish.

Developing an effective schedule can go a long way toward reaching your educational

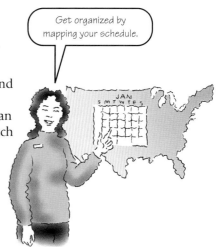

Get organized by mapping your schedule.

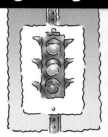

Signs & Signals

TIME MANAGEMENT TIPS

It can be hard to keep your focus when you're faced with a packed schedule. You might start to feel anxious about all the work that you have to do or tired and ready to throw in the towel. Follow these time management tips, and you'll stay on course toward your goals.

- Learn to discipline yourself, especially at the beginning and end of each term. Following a routine will help you stay disciplined and focus on your goal.
- Watch for study burnout. Avoid saving all of your studying for one night. Spread out your tasks throughout the week and get a good night's sleep. Pulling all-nighters will leave you exhausted and drained.
- Attend class regularly. This may seem obvious, but some students think they can miss class and still do well. If you skip class, you'll miss important information. If you must miss a class, arrange to get notes from a fellow student.
- Complete your homework on time. Homework is good practice and can help you work through information that you may not have fully understood in class.
- Review your goals and imagine what it will be like when you reach them. Visualizing doing well can give you the motivation to keep going!
- Be decisive. Make a pact with yourself that you'll accomplish something. After you complete a task, reward yourself.
- If you feel that you don't understand the material, don't be afraid to ask the instructor for assistance. Your instructor may even be able to suggest a tutor or study group that may be beneficial to you.
- Seek out support from family and friends if you start feeling overwhelmed.

goals. The most successful schedules include short-term and long-term planning. Your schedule should include the following:

- a general schedule for each term, including major assignments, tests and other key course dates, and personal dates/obligations

- a specific but flexible bi-weekly schedule
- a daily to-do list

You can use a calendar, journal, computer, or personal planner to help you create your schedule. It doesn't matter which tool you use, as long as you write (or type) it all down. Writing down activities, times, and dates will help you remember what needs to be done and to plan for it. Put your schedule in a place where you'll look at it often, such as on your desk or refrigerator. Although making a schedule may seem like extra work, being prepared and organized will make you more productive and efficient. In short, schedules make it easier for you to get things done!

Prioritize: First Things First

When you prioritize, you organize items by level of importance or urgency. Prioritizing your time means deciding how much time to devote to each of the various activities and obligations you must accomplish in a given day. When you have a lot to do in a short amount of time, it's always good to have a plan of action. The following steps will help you prioritize your time.

1. Make a list of everything you need to accomplish within a given time period. Your list can include your obligations as a student, as well as other social, personal, or work-related commitments.

2. Prioritize your daily to-do list. Decide which tasks you need to do first and which items you can save for later.

3. Think of each priority as a new goal, and then break each goal into smaller goals when necessary. For example, you might write, "I need to study the first three chapters before Friday's test. I'll study one chapter per night."

4. Be flexible. Your priorities may have to shift if deadlines change or if you add something new to your schedule.

To Do:
1. ~~Attend group meeting~~
2. ~~Study for Tuesday's quiz~~
3. Shop for groceries
4. Read Ch. 4 for Friday's Bio class
5. Pick up dry cleaning

Make a list of tasks and cross them off as you complete them.

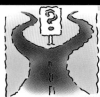

Fork in the Road

PRIORITIZING AND SCHEDULING

Make a list of at least five important things you'll need to accomplish by the end of next week. Then, organize the items on your list in order of priority. Label each item as "urgent" or "not urgent." Finally, create a schedule for the week by mapping out the days and times when you plan to accomplish each activity or task. For more complicated tasks, create several short-term goals leading up to their completion.

Avoid Procrastination Pitfalls

Procrastination means holding off for tomorrow what could be done today. Everyone procrastinates; it can become a hard habit to break. But procrastination leads to wasted time, missed opportunities, poor performance, and added stress. Individuals who procrastinate tend to place low-priority tasks before high ones in an attempt to avoid doing things they'd rather not do. They also tend to offer excuses for not completing high-priority tasks.

Do any of the following statements sound familiar?

- I'll wait until I'm in the mood.
- I'll think about it tomorrow.
- There's plenty of time to get it done.
- I don't know where to begin.
- I work best under pressure.
- I've got too many other things to do first.

Recognizing procrastination behavior and thinking is the first step toward putting a stop to it. The next time you find yourself avoiding a task and making excuses, follow these guidelines to give yourself a jump-start.

- If a task seems too large or intimidating, divide the work into smaller tasks. Completing several small tasks can give you the confidence and motivation you need to get the job done.
- Set realistic goals. Perfectionists sometimes find themselves procrastinating because they're afraid of not meeting their own unrealistic expectations. Give yourself a break and make sure your goals are achievable.
- Eliminate distractions. You may need to move to an area with fewer distractions so you can concentrate. Background

noise, such as the television, radio, or phone, can cause you to lose your focus.

- If you don't know where to start, seek out help from other sources. You may find it helpful to discuss the assignment with other students or your instructor. Doing research online or at the library is another way to get your ideas flowing.

> As Mark Twain said, "Do something every day that you don't want to do; this is the golden rule for acquiring the habit of doing your duty without pain."

Study Skills

Every successful student knows one thing: to master the material, you must first learn how to study. And successful students also know that there's more to studying than sitting down with a textbook and reading the assignment. Studying involves using techniques that help you learn and retain the information you need to know.

X Marks the Spot

When you study, you're behind the wheel, steering the course toward your goals. It's important that the course is as smooth as possible. You can't drive properly if a lot of distractions surround you. So, before you begin studying, you should find a calm, comfortable, and distraction-free environment. Choose two or three potential spots that you think might work for you. Then, ask yourself the following questions.

- Will I be comfortable in this space?
- Will I be interrupted by other people?
- Are there too many distractions, such as the television, phone, computer, or radio?
- Are the temperature and lighting okay? If not, can I adjust them?
- Can I use this space on a regular basis?

If the room or building is a public place, determine if it has been reserved for certain times or days. If the room is used for meetings or other gatherings, you may want to choose a place that's more readily available to you.

The Joy of Studying

When you think of fun and enjoyment, you might envision yourself going on a vacation, playing a game, or relaxing with your family or friends. The word "studying" probably doesn't come to mind. But studying can be a pleasant experience, if you allow it to be.

Studying gives you a chance to relax, think, and learn. As a student, you'll want to gain the maximum learning benefits from your study session. Here are a few suggestions to prepare your mind and body for studying.

- Add white noise to your study environment. Instrumental music, running water, or the sound of a whirring fan are all examples of white noise. White noise helps cover distracting sounds, such as traffic and talking.

- Play some soothing background music. A low level of background music can put you in a state of relaxed alertness, which increases learning. Music also triggers an emotional response that can be associated with a memory and can improve later recall.

- Get some exercise. Walking around or just doing some basic stretches before and during study sessions can help your brain learn and retain new information. Physical comfort is important for concentration.

Block outside distractions before studying so you can concentrate better.

STAY AWAY   DO NOT CROSS

Banishing Negative Thinking

Okay, you've found a spot to study in, you're comfortable, and you're ready to crack open that textbook. You take a peek at your schedule. You glance at the clock on the wall. You've got so much to do, and not a lot of time to accomplish everything. How are you going to get through all the required material before the big test? Suddenly, you feel overwhelmed, and you haven't even begun to study!

One of the biggest challenges to effective studying is getting started. It's easy to psych yourself out with negative self-talk. When you tell yourself you can't do something, you've already set yourself up to fail! Here are some examples of negative self-talk, and how to turn your doubts into encouragement.

Negative Self-Talk	Positive Affirmation
What's the point? I shouldn't even try.	I should try. If I don't try, I'll regret it later.
This is too hard.	This is hard, but I'm intelligent and capable. If I keep working, I'll eventually figure it out.
I can't do this.	I can do this, and I will do this!

A winning attitude helps you maintain a professional approach to your coursework. If you think you can succeed, then you will!

One Small Step at a Time

Have you ever heard the saying, "Rome wasn't built in a day"? It often takes time to make great things happen, so be patient with yourself. Large goals can seem too far off or unreachable. So, think big, but start small. Breaking up your large goal into smaller ones will make studying easier and large goals seem more attainable.

When determining how to study most efficiently, begin by asking yourself these questions.

- What do I want to get out of this study session?
- What do I need to know from the material?
- What's my goal? How am I going to break my goal into smaller goals?

If your goal is to read a chapter, begin by telling yourself that you'll read for 15 minutes. After 15 minutes, tell yourself you'll read for 15 more. When you see how far you've come, it will encourage you to keep reading.

Maintaining Your Focus

While you study, it's important to ask yourself reflective questions. Asking yourself questions about the text will keep you focused on what you're learning. If you don't know the answer to a question, it might mean that you've missed something important and you need to review that part again. The following questions are examples of reflective questions you can ask yourself while studying:

> As you read, ask yourself, "Why am I reading this?" and "What's important here?" These types of questions will help you stay focused.

- *Why am I reading or listening to this?* This will help you maintain your focus during the study session.

- *What's the overall content?* Skimming pages or reading introductory paragraphs will give you a bigger picture of the text and how much time you'll need to devote to each topic or section.

- *What's important here?* Not all of the information presented to you is of equal importance. Highlight key terms and ideas only. If you can't decide whether something is important, assume it is.

Taking Effective Notes

An important part of reading and studying is taking notes. Effective notes help you rephrase the material, giving you a better understanding of it. Your understanding of the material builds on itself. In some subjects, such as math, you need to fully understand each concept before you can move on. Taking notes helps you learn and remember the information more easily.

As you read, you can take notes by writing directly in your textbook or by using a separate sheet of paper. Whichever method you decide to use, follow these guidelines:

- Read each paragraph or section completely before marking or noting anything.
- If you had any questions about the material before you started reading, mark points that answer your questions or include these points in your notes.
- For items that appear in a series or sequence, create a numbered list. Numbered lists are especially helpful for remembering step-by-step processes.
- Identify any key terms, dates, places, and names.
- Write summaries of the main ideas in your notes or in the margins of your textbook. Also, include any questions or comments you may have about the material.
- If something is unclear or confusing, note it with a question mark. This will remind you to ask your instructor about it at the next class.
- Put a star by any material your instructor emphasizes in class and other extremely important information.
- Create a table of contents of important topics for each chapter you read.

Self-Test

After you've studied the material, test yourself. It's not always easy to know what you've absorbed and what you need to keep working on. Ask yourself the following questions about the information you've studied.

- *How can I paraphrase or summarize the information?* Putting the information in your own words will help you understand and remember it.
- *How can I organize the information?* Organizing text helps your brain categorize and group pieces of information together, helping you recall them later. Creating an outline is a great way to organize the information.
- *Can I associate the information with something familiar?* Associating new information with a song, rhyme, smell, or other environmental trigger will help you retain and recall the information later on.

- *How does the information fit with what I know?* Discovering how new information relates to what you already know can help you understand the big picture and make connections between different pieces of information.

K	W	L

You can use a K-W-L chart to help discover how new information relates to what you've already learned. Under "K," write all the information you already *know* about a particular subject. Under "W," write down what you *want to know* about the subject, and under "L," include what you *learn* from the new information.

Studying S.O.S.

If you start studying and find that you're confused or frustrated, ask your instructor for help. Instructors often post office hours, or times when they're available to meet with students one-on-one. If you're having difficulty, you might benefit greatly from meeting with your instructor outside the classroom to discuss the course material and ask further questions. Instructors are usually willing and happy to go over material and answer questions. They'll likely appreciate your motivation and work to encourage your success. Remember that instructors are there to help you, so take advantage of the opportunity to meet with them!

Test-Taking Strategies

The big test is approaching, and you can already feel the butterflies in your stomach. You've studied the material, but your anxiety is starting to get the best of you. What are you going to do?

The best way to conquer test-taking fears is to be well prepared. Thorough preparation includes:

- *Learning about the test.* Ask the instructor about the type of test (short answer, multiple choice, true-false, essay, etc.). If possible, review previous tests you've taken in the course to find out what to expect. Also, attend any review sessions offered by your instructor.
- *Creating a study plan.* Gather your review materials, such as your textbook, lecture notes, and any handouts from your

instructor. Then, create an organized plan for studying by setting goals for yourself. Develop a one-page study sheet, including only the most important topics and key terms.

On the day of the test, follow these general guidelines to ensure that you do your best.

- Get enough rest.
- Avoid caffeine, which can cause you to feel jumpy and negatively affect your concentration.
- Review your study sheet one last time.
- Bring all the supplies you'll need, including pens, pencils, extra paper, a calculator, and anything else allowed by your instructor.
- Arrive to class five to ten minutes early.
- Read all the instructions before starting the test.
- Budget your time during the test, taking into consideration the number of questions and the level of difficulty and point value of each.

The next sections provide specific strategies to help you tackle different types of tests.

Objective Tests

When taking an objective test, keep in mind that there can be only one correct answer to each question. Here are some tips for answering different types of objective test questions.

- *Multiple-choice questions.* There may be two or more answer choices that are partially correct. The key to mastering a multiple-choice test is to use the process of elimination to select the best, or most correct, answer. Sometimes, it helps to think of an answer before looking at the options.
- *True-false questions.* Some statements may be tricky—make sure a statement is entirely true or entirely false before choosing your answer. Also, watch out for "absolute" words, such as *all, always, never,* and *none.* These small words can add big meaning to true-false statements.
- *Short-answer questions.* When approaching a short-answer test, rank each test item according to level of difficulty. First, answer the questions you know. Next, tackle the questions you should be able to answer after a moment's thought. Finally, try to answer any remaining questions.
- *Problem-solving questions.* Again, solve the easiest problems first to get your brain warmed up. It's also important to show all your work—you may receive partial credit even if you

miscalculate something or make a simple mistake. If you get stuck, try using a different method to solve the problem.

Subjective Tests

In subjective (essay) tests, there can be more than one correct answer to each problem. You'll be graded on how well your essay demonstrates your understanding of the material. To complete this type of test successfully, follow these steps.

1. Read the directions, marking important words or phrases.

2. If the test provides a choice of several essay questions or topics, read each of them. Note any facts or thoughts that immediately come to mind and select the topic that generates the most information.

3. Keep your eye on the clock and plan how much time you'll need to write your essay. (This step is particularly important for tests that require you to write two or more essays.)

4. Organize your thoughts by creating an outline. Be sure to include an introduction, several points with supporting facts, and a conclusion.

5. Use your outline as a guide as you write the essay. Answer or restate the essay question in your introductory paragraph and make sure your conclusion sums up the point(s) you intended to make.

6. After you've finished writing, review your essay to make sure you followed directions and answered the question adequately. As you review your answer, also correct any spelling and grammar errors.

Ethics

Ethics applies to your daily activities as a student and will be equally important in the workplace. **Ethics** gives us guidelines for moral behavior and helps us determine the difference between what is considered "right" or "wrong."

For example, in school, ethics dictates that cheating on assignments or tests is wrong. By deciding that you'll do your own work when it comes to school assignments, you may be adhering to your own *personal ethics.* Your set of personal ethics is often influenced by your moral values and character traits. This set of ethics applies to everything you do, including school, work, and your personal interactions with people.

Medical ethics, on the other hand, relates to the specific principles that govern the behavior and conduct of health professionals. These principles define proper medical etiquette, customs, and professional courtesy. As a medical assistant, you'll be required to follow these principles.

PERSONAL ETHICS

A person's set of personal ethics is influenced in part by her character traits. All of us have character traits that make up who we are as individuals. We like many of the things about ourselves, and we'd probably like to change others. As a medical assistant, you'll find that some of your natural character traits will be beneficial when working with patients and coworkers, and other traits will need some refining or adjusting.

Understanding your character traits requires self-assessment. Look at the list of adjectives below. Which traits best describe you?

- honest
- kind
- patient
- courteous
- quick-tempered
- funny
- stubborn
- organized
- friendly
- reliable
- shy

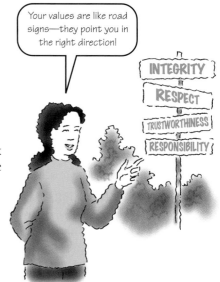

Your values are like road signs—they point you in the right direction!

INTEGRITY

RESPECT

TRUSTWORTHINESS

RESPONSIBILITY

Which ones did you choose? Can you think of more adjectives that describe you? Of the adjectives you chose, which do you think will prove helpful and which will you need to adjust to be an effective medical assistant? How do these traits relate to your own personal ethics? Read on to find out which values and character traits can help you become a successful medical assistant.

Integrity

Having **integrity** means that what you say and what you do are one and the same. When you have integrity, your actions reflect your inner ideals and ethics. Having integrity also means that

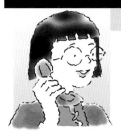

Ask The Professional

WHEN COWORKERS BEHAVE UNETHICALLY

Q: *I've noticed that one of my coworkers has been taking a lot of office supplies home. She'll take a ream of paper or a printer cartridge out of the supply cabinet and say that she'll replace it later when she has time to go to the office supply store. I've never actually seen her replace anything. She says she's too busy at work sometimes and isn't always able to run errands during the week. I know that taking office supplies isn't right, but is it really worth making a big deal about it? I'm afraid my coworker's attitude toward me will change if I tell a supervisor about what she's been doing.*

A: When you see coworkers cutting corners or disregarding rules in the medical office, you need to notify a supervisor. Although stealing office supplies may not seem like a big deal, the rule is there for a reason. Without office supplies, the medical office won't be able to meet the needs of its patients. And if staff members break other office rules, the consequences can be more serious. As a health care professional, it's important to have integrity and to abide by the rules even when they seem trivial. Patients are depending on you to provide quality care, which you'll be able to do if you're in the habit of doing the right thing, regardless of who is or isn't watching.

your behavior is consistent. A person with integrity behaves the same way from one situation to the next and doesn't make excuses when his actions are questioned.

Respectfulness

Everyone wants to feel respected. When we feel respected by someone, we feel important and deserving of that person's time and attention. As a medical assistant, it's especially important to treat everyone with respect, regardless of his status, position, educational level, or appearance. Respecting others includes the following behaviors:

- being courteous, including saying "please" and "thank you"
- addressing others by their proper titles
- acknowledging other people's feelings and concerns

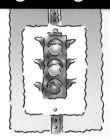

Signs & Signals

BUILDING GOOD RAPPORT

Rapport is the mutual feelings of trust and respect shared between people in a healthy relationship. Your goal as a medical assistant is to build good rapport with patients. The following tips will help you build good rapport with patients:

- Have a purpose and an objective for every interaction with a patient. If you're confused or disorganized, the patient may feel like you don't care about her time.

- The patient's needs should always be addressed. Be flexible, because a patient may wish to discuss something at length with you.

- Create a comfortable environment for the patient. An atmosphere that is relaxed and unhurried will encourage better communication between you and the patient.

- Communicate to the patient her confidentiality rights. A patient wants to feel that you're trustworthy when she's sharing private information with you. Failure to address this issue can be considered a breach of the patient's right to privacy.

- Observe a patient's gestures and facial expressions and respond accordingly. Paying attention to these clues makes you aware of the patient's feelings and concerns.

- Pace the conversation. Don't rush through an interaction with a patient, but let her know if time is limited.

- Respect the patient's personal space and be aware of how the patient responds to your presence.

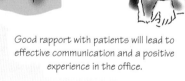

Good rapport with patients will lead to effective communication and a positive experience in the office.

- being tactful and sensitive in all dealings with people, including your coworkers, patients, and supervisor(s)
- choosing your words wisely

When it comes to respect, a good rule of thumb is: treat others the way you wish to be treated. Respecting yourself and those around you is one aspect of professional behavior.

Trustworthiness

Trustworthiness is another important quality to have as a medical assistant. Physicians and patients will rely on you to do an accurate and thorough job. A trustworthy employee is someone who is honest and reliable. He gives his word that something will be done, and then he does it.

A true professional is also honest in terms of admitting to his limitations. In the medical office, if you're unsure how to perform a task or procedure, ask a coworker to explain it to you. Being trustworthy doesn't mean that you take on every challenge by yourself, but rather that you have the good judgment to ask for help when you need it.

Likewise, it's important to be honest about any mistakes you make while working in the medical office. Some mistakes, such as giving the wrong medication, can be harmful to patients and should be reported to the physician immediately. Admitting to your mistakes is never easy, but having strong personal ethics will guide your actions in tough situations.

A person who takes responsibility is the captain of her own ship. She sets the course and actively pursues the journey.

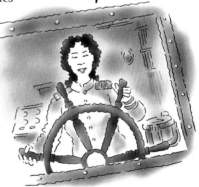

Responsibility

To be a successful medical assistant, your personal ethics need to include a strong sense of responsibility. Responsibility means:

- taking initiative in the workplace
- taking ownership in your profession and of your future career success
- taking pride in the work you do

Being a "Self-Starter"

If you have a strong sense of responsibility, you'll be committed to more than simply putting in a full day's work. Successful medical assistants are "self-starters." They take the initiative to seek out new work and information. A self-starter is proactive and makes things happen!

Taking Charge of Your Career

Taking ownership in your profession helps you work toward future career success and advancement. Taking ownership means that you feel responsible for the work you produce, and you care about quality and performance. You want to do the best job that you possibly can every single day that you're there.

People who take ownership of their careers get noticed. A supervisor is more likely to promote you if she really believes you care about the office as well as do your job well. Someone who takes ownership:

- admits to her mistakes
- doesn't make excuses
- plays fair
- fights for what she believes in
- accepts consequences
- is dedicated to doing a good job

Taking Pride in the Work You Do

Pride is the feeling we have when we know we've done a good job. By being an ethical and responsible worker, you help care for others and ensure their well-being. You should feel good about the work that you do! Taking pride in your work shows that you're dedicated to the profession and making strides toward bettering yourself as a medical professional.

MEDICAL ETHICS

Aside from your own personal ethics, you'll also be required to follow medical ethics as you perform daily tasks in the physician's office. The AAMA has developed specific ethical guidelines that medical assistants must follow. (You'll learn about the AAMA Code of Ethics in Chapter 7.) As a medical assistant, you'll be responsible for upholding medical ethics in all your duties, most importantly, in these two areas:

- patient advocacy
- patient confidentiality

Being a Patient Advocate

Being an advocate for patients means making sure their best interests are always placed first. In certain situations, you may need to set aside your own personal beliefs, values, or biases temporarily to provide the best care. However, it's important to keep in mind that being a patient advocate doesn't require you to take an action that would compromise your own value system.

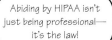

Abiding by HIPAA isn't just being professional—it's the law!

Protecting Patient Confidentiality

Another part of medical ethics is the importance of protecting patient confidentiality. In fact, it's not just ethical to keep patient information private—it's the law! The **Health Insurance Portability and Accountability Act (HIPAA)** is a federal law that determines how patients' medical information must be handled, stored, and transmitted. As a medical assistant, you will be responsible for handling patient information, so you'll need to be aware of the HIPAA rules that apply to the medical office.

For example, according to HIPAA, you must not release private patient information without the patient's consent. This means that even if a patient's family member calls the office requesting information, you must first obtain the patient's consent before providing confidential details about the patient's health. It also means that staff members shouldn't discuss patients' health conditions, because only those directly involved in a patient's care may have access to private health information.

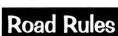

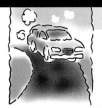

PROTECTING PATIENTS' RIGHTS UNDER HIPAA

Under HIPAA, patients have certain privacy rights. In the medical office, you can help protect these rights by knowing what they include:

- the right to give consent before information is released for treatment, payment, or health care operations
- the right to access their medical records
- the right to request that their medical records be amended for accuracy
- the right to be educated about the provider's policy on privacy protection
- the right to access the history of nonroutine disclosures
- the right to request that the provider restrict the use and routine disclosure of information the provider has, except in some legal and ethical situations.

Developing the Right Skills

You've likely developed many interesting skills over the years through your education and various jobs. You may be a skilled cook or piano player, or you may know how to solve any computer problem that comes along. You have likely also developed personal skills over the years, such as handling difficult social situations or making people feel at ease. Skillful people have learned and practiced an activity or task until they've mastered it and know how to solve problems when they arise. As a medical assistant, you'll need to be adept in the following skills:

- technical operations (using your hands)
- patient care skills
- communication
- patient education
- customer service
- critical thinking
- working as a member of a team

TECHNICALLY SPEAKING

You might not know it, but you use technical skills every day. When you perform basic tasks and operate simple machines, you are using your technical expertise. For example, driving is an operation that involves many technical skills. Steering the wheel, shifting gears, and adjusting the rearview mirror are all examples of technical skills required for driving safely.

What Are Technical Skills?

Technically skilled workers have the ability to use equipment skillfully to produce a desired outcome or result. Understanding how to use the equipment and materials in the medical office is part of professional behavior. Individuals who have good technical skills are able to:

- use manual dexterity and good hand-eye coordination
- troubleshoot when equipment malfunctions
- use equipment competently and with minimal trouble
- adapt equipment and technical procedures to meet the needs and challenges of all patients

Keep in mind, however, that technical skills aren't limited to the skills needed to operate equipment. They also include the technical skills you'll need to provide patient care. Laws governing the duties medical assistants perform vary from state to state. The tasks you may be asked to perform that require technical skills include:

- administering immunizations
- drawing blood specimens
- preparing and sterilizing instruments
- performing eye and ear irrigations
- obtaining vital signs (e.g., blood pressure, pulse, temperature)

Using Your Hands

Some people are naturally "good with their hands" and quickly develop competency with technical procedures. Others may have to practice procedures many times before being able to perform them correctly. Whatever your natural level of skill, you can master the manual skills necessary to becoming a successful medical assistant with patience and effort. The following tips will help you on your road to technical competency:

- Take time to familiarize yourself with the procedural equipment before using it with patients. Understand how it works and know the materials you'll need. If possible, anticipate problems and know how to remedy them.

- When a procedure requires dexterity, practice the necessary skill until you feel confident before attempting to perform it during a patient examination or treatment.

- Identify nurses and other professionals who are technical experts, and ask them to share their knowledge and experiences with you.

- Ask for help when you're feeling unsure about how to perform a procedure or manage equipment. A patient's well-being can depend on your good judgment.

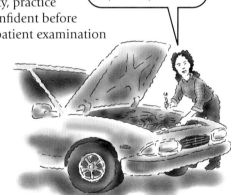

Technical skills are the tools we use to help solve patients' problems.

HITCH A RIDE ON THE COMMUNICATION EXPRESS

Good communication skills are an important part of working in a medical office. As a medical assistant, your duties will involve obtaining and providing accurate and thorough information. Learning and using effective communication techniques is part of becoming a professional in the medical field. The following

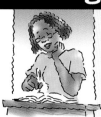

Travelog — GAINING TECHNICAL EXPERIENCE

As a student, I'm learning a lot about medical assisting—what skills I need to develop, what duties and responsibilities I'll have once I begin working in a medical office ... For the most part, it's exciting, but there are times when I worry about whether I'll be able to do certain things.

For instance, at first, I was apprehensive about some of the tasks I'd be asked to perform, especially giving injections. I felt unfamiliar with a needle and syringe and was afraid of hurting a patient if I inserted the needle improperly. We've read about different techniques in our textbooks, but it's hard for me to learn something new unless I have a chance to practice it. I talked to my instructor about my concerns, and he put my mind at ease. He reminded me that all students practice their technical skills in skills labs before they'll ever have to use those skills in the medical office. It's nice to know that I'll be able to perfect my technique before using it on an actual patient!

tips will help you communicate effectively with patients and coworkers.

- Think before you speak. A well-spoken, informed medical assistant presents a positive image to the patient and gains her trust and respect.
- Listen actively. Don't interrupt the speaker. Confirm that you've understood the message.
- Pay attention to clues. Our body language, facial expressions, and gestures often reflect our inner feelings. Be aware of these clues and respond accordingly.
- Use touch when it is appropriate. Touching a patient at the right moment can express your care and concern for her well-being.
- Give the patient enough space to feel comfortable. Standing or sitting too close to a patient when speaking can be intimidating.

Remember that professionalism requires strong communication skills, so it's important to learn what they are and how to use them. (Communication skills will be discussed in more detail in Chapter 2.)

PATIENT EDUCATION

Patient education is another key aspect of the professional medical assistant's job. You may be responsible for:

- explaining office policies and procedures to patients
- teaching good health habits and basic methods for disease prevention
- telling patients about local community resources, such as support groups suited to their specific needs
- providing instructions for taking medications prescribed by the physician
- educating patients about their newly diagnosed medical conditions

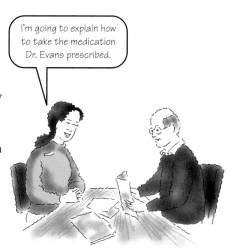

I'm going to explain how to take the medication Dr. Evans prescribed.

When educating patients in the medical office, it's important to convey information clearly and accurately. Strong communication skills will help you get the right message across. You may also need to adapt the information to the patient's level of understanding. (You'll learn tips to help you accomplish this in Chapter 4.)

Developing a Teaching Plan

When educating a patient, the first step you'll need to take is to develop a teaching plan. Make sure your teaching plan includes the following elements:

- *Learning goal.* What should the patient learn from this information?
- *Material to be covered.* What are the topics to be discussed?
- *Learning objective.* What steps or procedures need to be taken to ensure that the patient fully understands the material?
- *Evaluation.* How is the patient incorporating this information into his lifestyle?
- *Comments.* Are there any circumstances that might prevent the patient from completing the objectives successfully?

Developing New Material

For certain topics, the medical office may have resources and materials (such as pamphlets) already available. For other topics, you may need to develop new material. Follow these tips when developing new material for patient education.

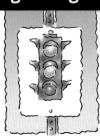

Signs & Signals — TEACHING TIPS

Here are a few general tips to help you provide effective patient education.

- Be aware of current medical issues, discoveries, and trends.
- Research special services available in your area.
- Keep relevant handouts and information sheets on hand.
- Allow enough time for the teaching session so you can avoid being interrupted or feeling rushed.
- If possible, take the patient to a quiet room to keep distractions to a minimum.
- Provide information in a clear, brief, step-by-step manner. Also, give the patient written instructions to take home.
- Give the patient enough time to process the information.
- Encourage the patient to ask questions or voice concerns.
- Gauge the patient's understanding of the material by asking questions.
- Instruct the patient to call the office with any additional questions.

- Indicate the objective of the information. What do you hope to accomplish by teaching this material to the patient?
- Personalize the information to capture the patient's interest. Explain to the patient how this information directly affects her life.
- Make sure all information is clear and well organized.
- Break up large chunks of information with lists and outlines.
- Avoid using medical jargon whenever possible.
- Use visual aids, such as diagrams and pictures that are clearly labeled and easy to follow.

CUSTOMER SERVICE: HOW MAY I HELP YOU?

Whenever you visit someplace new, whether it's a new school or a new city, you can feel like an outsider. A warm greeting, even if it's from a stranger, can put you at ease and make you feel welcome.

As a medical assistant, part of your job is to be that friendly face for patients. A visit to the medical office can make some patients anxious, so it's necessary to let patients know that they're safe and that their concerns are important to you.

Having good customer service skills involves serving patients and keeping their best interests at heart. On busy or stressful days, it can become difficult to convey a positive image to patients and staff. But it's important to retain a professional attitude and appropriate behavior at all times. The following tips, when put into practice, will help you achieve good customer service skills.

- Maintain a positive attitude. At times, patients may become angry or confused, and it's your job to remain calm in tense situations.
- Dress to impress. Looking your best will make you feel good about yourself, and others will feel good about you, too!
- Practice good personal hygiene.
- Be a role model. Take patient concerns seriously and address matters in a timely and efficient manner.
- Be courteous. Treat patients the way you'd like to be treated.
- Be diplomatic. Handle others with tact and genuine concern.

Remember that you only have one chance to make a first impression, so make it a good one. Good customer service skills and learning how to deal with patients are an important part of professionalism within the workplace. (You'll learn more about developing customer service skills in Chapter 3.)

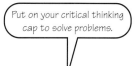

Put on your critical thinking cap to solve problems.

CRITICAL THINKING

Critical thinking is the ability to analyze problems and find reasonable solutions. One aspect of professionalism is the ability to think critically when there is a problem to solve in the medical office. Strong critical thinking skills will help you provide effective care to patients. Critical thinking also helps you troubleshoot potential problems to maintain an efficient office.

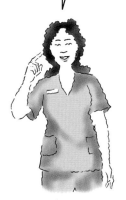

Smart Thinking

Medical assistants with strong critical thinking skills are able to do the following:

- understand potential problems and consequences
- solve problems creatively
- brainstorm solutions

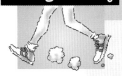

Running Smoothly

MAINTAINING A GOOD ATTITUDE

What if a patient becomes angry or irritated?

A patient you're speaking with over the phone is becoming increasingly irritated. He wants to make an appointment during a time when the physician will be seeing patients in the hospital. You explain to him that the physician will be at the hospital at that time. The patient says angrily, "It's impossible to get an appointment with this office! You people don't know how to do your jobs!" How do you handle a situation like this?

Patients who are ill or who are worried about their condition can become irritable or upset. In these situations, it's important to have self-control and maintain a professional attitude. Instead of arguing with the patient, try to calm him and communicate your desire to help without sounding patronizing. You may say something like, "I understand your concern, Mr. Smith. Let me take a look at the schedule to see if we can find another appointment time that is convenient for you."

- choose solutions that are most likely to produce the desired outcomes
- use the critical thinking method

The Critical Thinking Method

You can use the critical thinking method when you've been posed with a thinking challenge. To answer the challenge, follow these five steps.

1. Identify the purpose, or goal, of your thinking. This will help you direct all your thoughts toward that goal. For example, your goal might be to decide which action to take in a given situation.

2. Determine whether the knowledge you have is accurate, complete, and relevant. Where did you receive the information? Is your source reliable, or do you need to investigate the situation yourself?

3. Spot potential problems that can cloud your reasoning. As you learn to think critically, this will become

easier to do. Problems include working with faulty assumptions, accepting unproven arguments, being biased, or allowing emotion to interfere with your reasoning.

4. Seek out helpful resources. Professionals are quick to recognize their limitations and seek help from other sources, such as experienced coworkers, texts and journals, and office policies or guidelines.

5. Critique your judgment or decision. Identify alternative judgments and weigh the benefits and possible consequences of each option. Then, reach a conclusion.

After using the critical thinking method to solve a problem or make a difficult decision, assess how well you used the method. Use the standards for critical thinking to judge your performance. Critical thinking should be:

- clear
- precise
- specific
- accurate
- relevant

Road Rules   USING THE CRITICAL THINKING METHOD

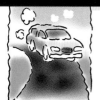

Using the critical thinking method can be challenging; it requires you to organize your thoughts and judge them according to a set of standards. Remember the following key information to help you use the critical thinking method effectively.

- Use the critical thinking method when you're posed with a thinking challenge. In other words, use it when there is a problem that calls for a resolution.

- Be sure to follow all five steps of the critical thinking method: identify your goal, assess the information you have, identify potential problems, seek out helpful resources, and critique your judgment or decision.

- During critical thinking, critique or judge your thoughts according to the standards for critical thinking.

- plausible (it should make sense)
- consistent
- logical
- deep
- broad
- complete
- significant
- adequate (for the purpose or goal you had in mind)
- fair

Getting in the Right State of Mind

If you want to think critically, you have to get into the right state of mind. Establishing specific thinking habits will train your mind to think critically. Incorporating the following tips into your thinking process will help you become a critical thinker.

- Think independently. Don't let others influence your decisions.
- Be fair-minded. Consider all sides of an argument before coming to a decision.
- Know when to ask for help. Admit when you've made a mistake or don't know something.
- Be intellectually courageous. Take chances, even when your thoughts are unpopular or challenging to others.
- Demonstrate good faith and integrity. Avoid letting bias cloud your judgment.
- Be curious and keep at it! Refuse to accept easy answers; instead, keep questioning until you're satisfied that you've looked at a situation from every angle.
- Be disciplined. Take the time you need to reach a sound conclusion. You may need to obtain additional information or seek advice from experienced coworkers before making a decision.
- Think creatively. Brainstorming can help you "think outside the box" to discover possible solutions.
- Have confidence in yourself! Once you learn to think critically, you'll have more confidence in your decisions. When questioned by a patient or coworker, you can stand by your decision and explain your reasons for making it.

TEAM PLAYERS WANTED

Teamwork is an important part of any medical office. Every member of the medical staff works together as a team to accomplish the same goal. Working together can improve:

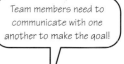

Team members need to communicate with one another to make the goal!

- efficiency in the office
- rapport with patients and between members of the health care team
- the quality of care provided to patients

Good teamwork includes the following elements:

- Everyone understands their personal responsibilities.
- Team goals are clear.
- Everyone takes some responsibility for leadership.
- Everyone actively participates.
- Everyone shows respect for one another.
- Everyone feels appreciated and supported.
- Team members listen to each other.
- Different opinions are respected.

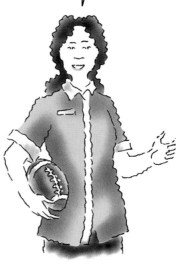

Road Rules   WORKING TOGETHER

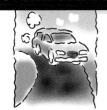

Working together can be a challenge, but it can also be fun! Communicating with others and sharing the same tasks helps build strong working relationships. Getting along with your coworkers makes it easier to work well with them. Remember to keep in mind the following tips about working together.

- Working together to reach a desired goal requires good teamwork.
- Working well together can improve *efficiency, rapport,* and the *quality of care* provided to patients.
- In a team, everyone feels supported and appreciated.
- A team player knows what his personal responsibilities are.

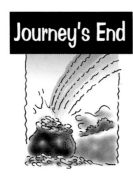

Journey's End

- Professionalism is the attitude of being a professional, that is, of having a positive outlook and a commitment to doing your best at all times.

- As you acquire the education, ethics, and skills that make up the different aspects of professionalism, you'll be further on your journey toward becoming a successful medical assistant.

- You can learn to be a successful student by developing and using the right study and test-taking skills. To study effectively, choose a distraction-free study area, divide large tasks into smaller steps, and test your knowledge to see how much you've learned. To do well on tests, make sure you're adequately prepared and use specific strategies, such as reading all the directions before beginning and budgeting your time wisely during the test.

- Successful medical assistants possess integrity and are respectful and trustworthy.

- By using self-assessment, you can identify your own character traits. Some of these traits may be helpful to your future career as a medical assistant, whereas other traits may warrant changes.

- It's important for medical assistants to demonstrate responsibility because patients often rely on their care.

- Showing initiative in the workplace means that you're a "self-starter," or someone who continually seeks out work and additional information.

- The critical thinking method includes five steps: identifying your goal, assessing the information you have, identifying potential problems, seeking out helpful resources, and critiquing your judgment or decision.

- Learning how to think critically as a student will prepare you for the problem-solving situations you'll face in a medical office setting.

- Team-playing skills include carrying out your own responsibilities (pulling your own weight), listening to other team members and respecting their opinions, and working with others toward a clear goal.

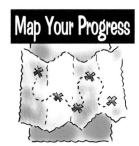
Map Your Progress

Answer the following multiple-choice questions.

1. Why should you break large goals into smaller ones?
   a. so that you become a professional
   b. so that you aren't overwhelmed
   c. so that you aren't bored
   d. so that you stay involved

2. *Rapport* is:
   a. the motivation to work toward achieving your goals.
   b. the ability to think critically.
   c. the mutual feelings of trust and respect shared between people.
   d. the ability to ensure patient confidentiality.

3. *HIPAA* stands for:
   a. Health Insurance Portability and Accountability Act.
   b. Health Information Privacy Protection Act.
   c. Health Insurance Protection for the Aged Act.
   d. none of the above

4. What is *not* part of a good first impression?
   a. practicing good hygiene
   b. greeting a patient with a friendly smile
   c. talking about your personal problems with a patient
   d. having a positive attitude

5. Why is it important to be a team player?
   a. Working well with others allows you to provide better patient care.
   b. Working well with others allows you to make more friends.
   c. Working well with others makes you popular and well liked.
   d. Working well with others improves your technical skills.

6. What does it mean to be a "self-starter"?
   a. You are content in your job.
   b. You are proactive and take initiative.
   c. You are honest in all your actions.
   d. You make a good first impression.

7. Having *integrity* means that you:
   a. are tactful and sensitive in all your dealings with people.
   b. take ownership of your future career success.
   c. display actions that reflect your inner ideals and ethics.
   d. take the initiative to seek out new work and information.

8. When using the critical thinking method, your first step should be to:
   a. seek out helpful resources, such as experienced coworkers.
   b. spot potential problems that can cloud your reasoning.
   c. identify alternative judgments and weigh the benefits of each option.
   d. identify the purpose, or goal, of your thinking.

9. What is *accreditation?*
   a. a required educational course for medical assisting students
   b. a process that evaluates educational programs for quality based on academic and administrative standards
   c. a standard examination given to medical assisting students upon graduation
   d. an evaluation of each student's technical skill level

10. Setting goals and focusing on them can help you:
    a. rely on a support system.
    b. stay motivated.
    c. remain calm.
    d. develop personal ethics.

Chapter 2

TAKING FLIGHT WITH COMMUNICATION SKILLS

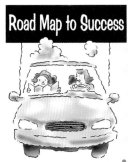

Road Map to Success

- Explain the importance of proper and effective verbal communication skills when encountering patients and coworkers
- Describe effective active listening skills
- List the topics that are covered in new patient interviews
- Describe the process for updating information when interviewing established patients
- Define therapeutic communication
- Explain the importance of therapeutic communication within a health care setting
- Explain the importance of teamwork within a health care setting
- Demonstrate how to use office communications equipment properly

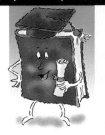

Chapter Competencies

- Recognize and respond to verbal and nonverbal communication (ABHES 2.i., ABHES 2.k., ABHES 2.l., CAAHEP 3.c.1.b., CAAHEP 3.c.1.c.)
- Interview effectively (ABHES 2.f.)
- Document appropriately (CAAHEP 3.c.2.d.)
- Be a "team player" (ABHES 1.c.)
- Serve as a liaison between the physician and others (ABHES 2.d.)
- Use proper telephone techniques (ABHES 2.e., CAAHEP 3.c.1.d.)

- Use correct grammar, spelling, and formatting techniques in written works (ABHES 2.j.)

- Demonstrate fundamental writing skills (ABHES 2.0.)

You probably don't think about it, but you communicate every day. When you say "hello," write an e-mail, or even smile at someone else, you are communicating a message. When you listen to someone and give advice or information, you are communicating. Communication is the tool we use to relate to and understand one another.

In this chapter, you'll learn valuable communication skills to use in the medical office. By learning how to communicate effectively with supervisors, coworkers, and patients, you'll be further on your way toward becoming a professional medical assistant.

Communication 101: The Basics

Communication requires at least two people.
- The *sender* is the person talking.
- The *receiver* is the person listening.

Communication involves two people actively sharing the roles of sender and receiver. Communicating with someone is like taking a journey together. When you're traveling and get lost, you stop and ask for directions. When someone communicates a message and you're confused, you ask him to clarify the message. What is the conversation's destination, and how are you going to get there?

- You seek **clarification,** or an explanation, when you're confused by someone's message.

- You give **feedback** by acknowledging that you understand the information the person is communicating. You can give feedback by saying, "Yes, I understand," or simply by nodding in agreement.

As a medical assistant, you'll communicate with patients and coworkers on a daily basis. Learning to use good communication skills is an essential part of becoming a successful medical assistant. Your communication will primarily focus on information pertaining to office policies and procedures and patient care. To ensure that you communicate accurately and properly, your tasks will include the following:

- conveying accurate information in a straightforward and clear manner

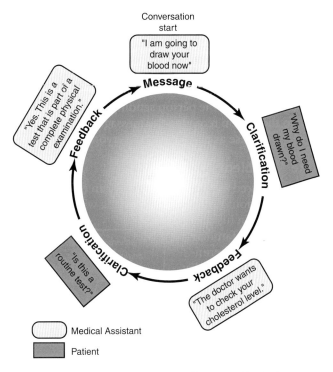

Conversation
start

"I am going to
draw your
blood now"

Message

"Why do I need
my blood
drawn?"

Clarification

Feedback

"Yes. This is a
test that is part of a
complete physical
examination."

Clarification

"Is this a
routine test?"

Feedback

"The doctor wants
to check your
cholesterol level."

Medical Assistant

Patient

Good communication involves clarification and feedback.

- clarifying messages when a person seems unsure or confused
- listening actively to obtain accurate information
- asking for clarification when you're unsure what someone else is trying to communicate
- giving feedback to show the other person that you understand the message being communicated
- asking for feedback to make sure the message you sent was received as intended

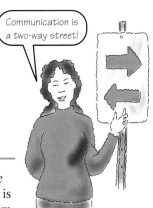

Communication is a two-way street!

Verbal Communication Skills

Verbal communication involves using words or language to convey a message. Most often, verbal communication is spoken. In the medical office, you'll need good verbal communication skills when:

- making appointments over the phone
- talking with patients in the office
- sharing information with the physician and other office staff

THE POWER OF WORDS

When speaking with patients, be sure to use language they'll easily understand. Using unnecessarily large words may distract or confuse a patient, and your meaning may not make as strong an impact.

Remember that the person sending a message has an obligation to the person receiving the message, and vice versa. Be as clear and precise as possible, and everyone will be understood.

Sounds Like "Gobbledygook" to Me!

Using advanced medical terminology can frighten a patient and cause confusion. When communicating with a patient, try putting yourself in his place. He may not be familiar with the medical terminology you use every day. You'll need to communicate in layman's terms so each patient is able to understand the message you're trying to convey.

> . . . atherosclerosis . . . angina pectoris . . . myocardial infarction . . .

> It sounds like "gobbledygook" to me!

Proper and Professional

When speaking to a patient, you should always use proper English and grammar. Relying on slang, even when you're stressed or in a hurry, presents an unprofessional image. Think about the difference between how you communicate with your friends and how you communicate with your instructors. When you're talking with friends, it's fine to use more informal language. But when speaking with an instructor, you should be polite and professional and use proper English and grammar. In a professional setting, speak to everyone—patients, coworkers, and physicians—with the same respect you would give to an instructor.

PARALANGUAGE

It's not only what you say, but how you say it, that makes all the difference. How you say something is called **paralanguage,** which includes several elements of your voice, such as:

- tone
- quality
- volume

- pitch
- range

Using appropriate paralanguage can help you emphasize a point or express a feeling. For example, if your voice has a sarcastic tone or your phrases are mumbled, a patient might feel like you don't care or are rude. However, if your voice is calm and sympathetic, the patient is more likely to trust you to do what is best for her. Using paralanguage that is appropriate and considerate is an essential part of good patient care.

It's important that you're aware of your own paralanguage. Do you sometimes speak too softly? Do friends joke about your tendency to say things very quickly? When talking with patients and coworkers, you must consider the words you say and how you are sending these messages.

THE SOUNDS WE MAKE

Nonlanguage sounds offer clues to how a person is feeling. Examples of nonlanguage sounds include:

- laughing
- sighing
- sobbing
- grunting

Be very aware of the sounds people make. Some patients may be hesitant to say what is wrong, but their nonlanguage sounds can convey important messages. It's essential to listen for these sounds when examining a patient. For example, if you're examining a patient and she makes an "ouch" sound, this nonlanguage clue tells you she is in pain. Asking a question such as "Did that hurt you?" will help clarify the patient's problem. It will also let her know that you're aware of her needs and you want to help.

Written Communication Skills

As a medical assistant, you will spend much of your time talking to patients and physicians. However, written communication is just as important in the medical office. Written communication involves using written language to exchange messages. Written communication can take the form of:

- e-mails
- letters
- prescriptions
- patient records

As a medical professional, your writing should always be clear and concise—and the content should always be accurate. Written information or instructions often serve as a reminder or reinforcement of what was previously discussed with a patient. If information or instructions aren't expressed clearly, the patient's medical care and treatment could be negatively affected. It's even possible for a patient to sue a medical office for poorly communicated written instructions. To protect patients and your medical office, be sure to communicate written information accurately, completely, and clearly. In addition, record and copy all important information and documents.

KEEP IT SIMPLE

When giving written instructions to a patient, it's important to keep it simple. Choose your words carefully, just as you would if you were speaking to the patient. Provide the necessary information, but use language the patient will understand. Here are some guidelines to follow when using written communication to instruct a patient.

- Take the time to write neatly. A patient may not understand what you have written because it's simply illegible.
- Take the time to ensure that the instructions are complete and accurate.
- Use proper spelling and grammar. Using slang or incorrect grammar presents an unprofessional image.
- Be sure to use language that is simple but clear and specific.

Written instructions should be clear to prevent confusion.

For example, a written message such as "Come back to the office if you don't feel better" isn't specific. It doesn't provide enough information or give clear instructions. Better instructions would be: "If your fever and sore throat aren't better in 24 hours, contact the office to schedule a second appointment." Sending a clear message to the patient will help prevent confusion or misunderstanding.

Giving written instructions to a patient is a form of patient education. When you're educating a patient about his condition or treatment plan, remember that in addition to written communication skills, verbal and nonverbal skills are also important. Using a variety of skills will help you communicate the clearest and most accurate message possible.

ASK QUESTIONS

When you give a written message to a patient in person, it's important to make sure the patient understands your message. A good way to check that the patient understands is to ask a follow-up question or to restate the information verbally. Be aware of the patient's body language. Ask yourself:

- Is he nodding?
- Does he seem to be fully engaged with the conversation?
- Does he seem puzzled or unresponsive?

(See *Understanding Body Language.*)

Remember to be tactful in your approach. You don't want patients to feel as if you're talking down to them. Remember, most patients don't have the medical knowledge that you do and may not understand exactly what you're saying. Following up and asking questions will help you avoid the misunderstandings that can sometimes occur with written communication.

WHEN IN DOUBT, WRITE IT OUT!

When writing messages or taking notes, think about the person who will be receiving the message. Using common medical abbreviations or shorthand may be acceptable when you're communicating with the physician or other office staff members. But keep in mind that patients may not understand these abbreviations. If you're ever unsure whether the person receiving the message will understand an abbreviation's meaning, write out the entire word or phrase instead. This will ensure accuracy in your written communication.

Nonverbal Communication Skills— Now You're Talking!

By now you know that speaking and writing help convey a message to another person. But did you know that what you *don't* say can be just as meaningful as what you *do* say? Nonverbal skills are a very important part of face-to-face communication. Nonverbal communication skills include:

- body language
- sensitivity to personal space
- the use of touch

If you don't give nonverbal clues when you speak, others will find it difficult to understand the meaning of your words.

> Nonverbal messages are the "tour guides" that help you communicate more easily.

UNDERSTANDING BODY LANGUAGE

Be aware of the physical messages you express when communicating. Your words may say one thing, but your body may say something entirely different. If your verbal message doesn't match your nonverbal message, a patient may suspect that you are lying or lacking integrity. Your body language can make a lasting impression on patients—you want to make sure it's a positive one!

Kinesics refers to body movements, which can include:

- facial expressions
- gestures
- eye movements

Kinesics often reveal how a person is feeling.

Your body language should be just as positive as your verbal language. For example, if you nod and smile at patients

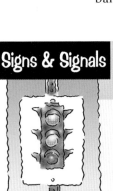

Signs & Signals

READING THE SIGNS: PATIENTS' BODY LANGUAGE

Patients may convey messages with body language. When patients are worried or upset, those feelings might show on their faces. It never hurts to ask patients how they're feeling. This makes patients feel validated; they're reassured that you're aware of them and care about their health.

When communicating with patients, it's also important to pay attention to whether their verbal messages match their nonverbal messages. For example, suppose a patient tells you, "I feel fine. My back pain hasn't been that bad recently." However, his body language suggests otherwise: the patient keeps his hand on his back and winces slightly when he gets up from the examination table. Because patients sometimes mask their feelings, you'll need to recognize inconsistent messages and adjust your care accordingly.

while they are talking, they're more likely to believe that you're truly engaged and listening. But what if you nod and smile while repeatedly glancing at the clock during a conversation? Patients might think you don't care about what they have to say. If patients don't feel that you care about them and their health, they are less likely to feel confident under your care.

GIVE ME SPACE!

By now you understand that when communicating with others, what you say is just as important as how you say it. Did you know that where you say it is another important factor in communicating?

Proxemics refers to the physical space between two people who are communicating. Imagine a sphere around yourself that extends about three feet outward; this is your "personal space." This means you probably allow at least three feet between yourself and the person you're communicating with. Everyone requires some amount of personal space during a conversation, and the amount can vary depending on personality and culture. Unwanted intrusion into an individual's personal space can cause him to feel uncomfortable, angry, or even threatened.

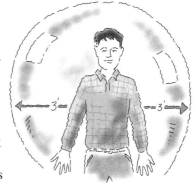

Most people require about three feet of "personal space."

As a medical assistant, you'll need to enter a patient's personal space to provide care and treatment. It's important to approach a patient professionally and to explain to him what you're about to do. This will help ease the patient into the treatment or procedure.

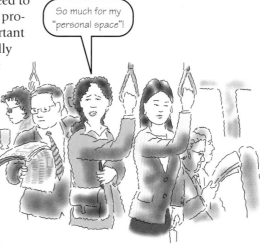

So much for my "personal space"!

After the patient has been treated, it's good to take a step back to allow for more space between yourself and the patient. This may help him feel more comfortable and in control. Whenever you're communicating with a patient, you always want to make him feel as comfortable as possible.

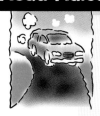

Road Rules   THE RULES OF BODY LANGUAGE

- How you say something, or *paralanguage*, affects the message you're trying to communicate.
- *Nonlanguage* sounds give insight into how a patient is feeling.
- Your body language, or *kinesics*, should be just as positive as what you say.
- Be aware of *proxemics*, a patient's required personal space, when communicating.

Communicating with Patients

There are a variety of important skills to use when communicating with patients. When you travel, you want the journey to be smooth and efficient. An easy journey makes the ride or flight a positive experience. When you communicate professionally, you want your conversations to be positive experiences for patients. And patients want you to hear and understand them. How are you going to do that for them? Read on to find out!

LISTEN WITH YOUR WHOLE BODY

As a medical professional, it's important to know when you should speak and when you should listen. **Active listening** means you are mentally and physically engaged with what the other person is saying. Your full attention is on the other person, and you are listening and watching for verbal and nonverbal clues.

How do you let a patient know that you're actively listening to her? Here are some active listening tips.

- Turn your body toward the speaker.
- Make eye contact.
- Rephrase the information to let the speaker know that you understand.
- Ask questions when you are confused.

Glancing around the room or giving a blank facial expression will show the speaker that you aren't fully engaged with the conversation. In fact, poor listening can even affect the quality of care you provide to the patient. Would you ignore a road

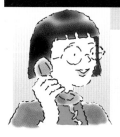

Ask The Professional

LISTENING ACTIVELY TO AVOID MISCOMMUNICATION

Q: *Last week, when I was talking with Mr. Lee and recording information in his medical chart, I remembered that I forgot to return another patient's phone call. I was so worried about calling this patient that I became distracted and wrote something incorrect on Mr. Lee's chart. Confusing his medical needs with the needs of the other patient, I scheduled him for the wrong type of test. Luckily, the physician spotted my error, but Mr. Lee was furious. How can I avoid these types of miscommunications in the future?*

A: It's always important to listen actively to the patient with whom you're speaking and focus on the task at hand. Otherwise, you may end up making an error that could cause harm to the patient. Of course, unexpected situations will arise and you need to be flexible. The next time you remember something important, politely excuse yourself and make a note so that you don't forget about the task. That way, you'll be able to devote all your attention to the current patient or task, instead of the tasks that you've yet to complete.

sign if it was pointing you in the right direction? Listening to the patient will let her know that you value her thoughts and concerns, which will help you on your journey to success as a medical assistant.

PATIENT INTERVIEWS

As a medical assistant, you may be responsible for gathering information about new patients and updating information about current patients. This task is done by interviewing each patient. The new patient interview covers a range of topics, including:

- *Past medical history.* Does the patient have any chronic medical problems (e.g., diabetes or heart disease)? Has the patient ever been hospitalized before?

- *Family health history.* Are there any genetic disorders in the patient's family (e.g., certain cancers or some forms of high blood pressure)? Do the patient's parents suffer from any health problems? If the patient's parents are deceased, what was the cause of death and at what age did they die?

- *Body systems review.* Is the patient having problems with any of the major body systems (cardiovascular, neurological, immune, etc.)?

- *Social history.* Does the patient smoke? What is the patient's occupation? What are the patient's hobbies?

- *Medications.* Is the patient currently taking any medications, vitamins, or herbal supplements?

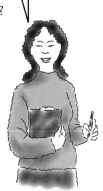

When documenting patient information for the physician, remember the three most important things: accuracy, accuracy, accuracy!

The goal of this first interview is to obtain accurate and thorough information regarding the new patient. If the patient seems uncomfortable answering certain questions, explain to the patient that this information will help the physician provide proper treatment and care. For this reason, it's also important to document the patient's responses clearly and completely. The physician will need accurate and thorough information to make diagnoses and develop appropriate treatment plans.

The interviewing procedure for an established patient is quite different. Follow these steps when updating information about a current patient.

1. First, review the patient's chart to familiarize yourself with the patient's health problems.

2. Next, make a list of questions pertaining to the patient's medical problems and any other concerns or discrepancies you find.

3. Then, ask the patient to state his chief complaint, or reason for the office visit. Accurately and thoroughly document any symptoms the patient has been experiencing.

4. Finally, reconfirm that the patient is currently taking the medications listed on his chart and ask him if he is undergoing any specific treatments that aren't listed.

The following sections describe the communication skills you can use to conduct successful patient interviews.

Reflecting on the Details

Reflecting is repeating what the patient said, using open-ended phrases or questions. You begin a sentence, but allow the patient to finish it. For example, you might say, "Mrs. Garcia, you said that when your stomach hurts you . . ." Reflection lets the patient make a more detailed response. It also helps you refocus the conversation when it has begun to drift to other subjects.

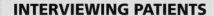 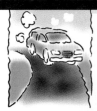

Road Rules — INTERVIEWING PATIENTS

- Make a list of the questions you need to ask, and be organized.
- Respect the patient's personal information by conducting the interview in a private area.
- Listen actively. Give the patient your full attention by looking and listening for verbal and nonverbal clues.
- Record accurate and detailed notes. The physician relies on the information in a patient's chart when diagnosing conditions and prescribing treatments.
- Remember that you are often the first person a patient meets, so you must demonstrate a professional and pleasant attitude at all times.

Reflecting is a useful skill, but be careful not to overuse it. Some patients may feel annoyed or patronized when you repeat their words back to them too often.

It's also important to allow a patient to finish speaking before taking notes. By writing notes as the patient is speaking, you may miss vital details. If there is a lot of information to document, politely ask the patient to pause for a moment so you can catch up on your notes.

So You Were Saying . . .

Paraphrasing is restating what you have heard, using your own words. Paraphrasing can help you verify that you have accurately heard and understood the information presented. It also gives a patient time to clarify what he has said. A paraphrased statement might sound like this: "I'd like to make sure I understand. You are saying that . . ." or "It seems like . . ." followed by the paraphrased information.

May I Have an Example, Please?

When you're confused or need further explanation from a patient, ask the patient to give an example of the situation. If a patient's description is vague, you might ask, "Can you give me an example of what happened when your symptoms occurred?" Asking for clarification will help you better understand the patient's needs. It also will let you know how a patient perceives the problem.

What? When? How?

Asking open-ended questions will help you gather specific information from a patient. Open-ended questions are the "what," "when," and "how" questions. Some examples include:

- "What symptoms have you been experiencing?"
- "When did you start experiencing pain?"
- "How did you burn your arm?"

Be careful when asking "why" questions because these kinds of questions might sound judgmental or accusatory. For example, asking, "Why did you do that?" or "Why didn't you do what the doctor said?" might make the patient feel upset, and she could become defensive or uncooperative. You want the patient to feel comfortable telling you her full story. Therefore, you might ask, "Is there something I need to explain more clearly?" This reminds the patient that you're on her side and are there to help.

Avoid using closed-ended sentences that allow the patient to answer in one word, such as "yes" or "no." You may not receive all the relevant information from a patient. For example, if you ask, "Are you eating at regular intervals during the day?" the patient may simply give a brief answer, such as "Yes." However, if you say, "Tell me what time you typically eat your meals," the patient will give a more specific description of his daily routine. The more information you obtain, the better you can treat the patient.

Sum It All Up

After you've gathered information from the patient, you'll want to review briefly what the patient has told you. **Summarizing**

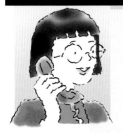

Ask The Professional   GETTING ALL THE FACTS

Q: *I was updating a patient's chart the other day, but I was having a hard time gathering the information I needed. Every time I asked a question, the patient would give me one-word answers. What did I do wrong?*

A: When you need to gather specific information about a patient's symptoms or condition, use open-ended questions. Ask a question that can't be answered with a simple "yes" or "no." For example, instead of asking, "Has the pain been severe?" say, "Please describe the pain you've been experiencing."

the information to the patient allows her to correct any miscommunications or add important details that you might have missed the first time. Summarizing can also help you organize and condense complicated information into a sequential order. For example, you might use words such as:

- *first*
- *then*
- *next*

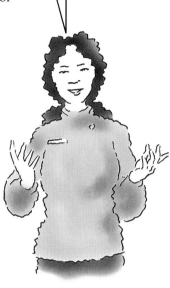

Summarizing lets the patient know that you have listened and understood what she told you.

THERAPEUTIC COMMUNICATION

Therapeutic communication uses certain verbal and nonverbal skills to increase the overall quality of patient care. Therapeutic communication is meant to convey a feeling of **empathy,** or concern for and understanding of a patient's feelings and sense of well-being. Therapeutic skills include:

- allowing time for silences
- knowing when and how to touch a patient
- using humor to relieve tension and stress
- using appropriate body language, including facial expressions that show concern

Knowing these skills and how to use them will help you become a successful and effective medical assistant.

Don't Be Afraid of Silence

Silence is often an overlooked and undervalued part of therapeutic communication. For some people, silence can be uncomfortable and even stressful. They may try to break the silence in an effort to keep the conversation moving along. But for others, silence is a welcome and necessary part of any conversation. Whatever the case may be, you shouldn't be afraid of silence when communicating with patients.

Periods of silence allow patients to:

- gather their thoughts
- assess their feelings
- recall information

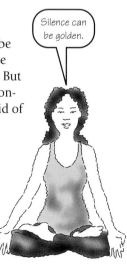

Silence can be golden.

You can use moments of silence as well. They give you time to process the information you've just heard and form more questions.

What's the Cause?

It's important to gauge how the patient is feeling so you can try to determine the cause for the patient's silence. Periods of silence can occur for a variety of reasons (positive and negative), such as:

- The patient is comfortable with silence. Excessive talking is unnecessary and intrusive.
- The patient needs some time to think and process how he's feeling.
- The patient is fearful of the procedure or treatment.
- The patient wants to show emotional strength or resilience.
- The patient feels angry and is using silence to express this emotion.

Creating a Comfort Zone

As a medical assistant, you should always strive to make the patient as comfortable as possible. You might choose to discuss the silence with the patient to understand its meaning better. Then you'll know the appropriate way to respond. For example, you might say, "Mrs. Davis, I know this might be painful to talk about. Please take all the time you need to gather your thoughts." This will help put the patient at ease. It might also give her the courage to express the reason for her silence.

However, while it's important to create a comfort zone for the patient, it's also necessary to avoid making offensive or misleading statements. For example, it would be misleading to say, "Everything is going to be all right" to a patient who is terminally ill. Such statements are not only misleading; they can also seem insincere. In these situations, it's better to listen to the patient and try to understand her concerns instead of saying something that may not be true.

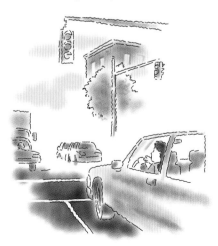

Less Talking, More Listening

Excessive talking can fluster a patient, especially if you ask too many questions. Be patient. Allow time for the patient to respond. It's important to be personable, but too much talking can take the focus away from the patient, where it needs to be.

Wait for the "green light" on communication.

It can also be helpful to remind the patient why you need to ask the questions you're asking. By reassuring patients that you're concerned with helping the physician provide the best care, they may feel more comfortable sharing their private medical concerns.

The Healing Touch

Just as a kind word can improve someone's day, a gentle touch can be an effective way to communicate warmth and compassion toward a patient. Touch is a powerful therapeutic tool that can help a patient in many ways, such as:

- providing reassurance
- helping a patient feel less lonely
- building a patient's self-esteem
- providing emotional support

But a patient also can perceive touch as threatening, hostile, or invasive. It's important to know when touching a patient is appropriate and how to do it effectively.

How to Use Touch

Touch can communicate comfort to a patient, but it also can be perceived negatively. Therefore, it's necessary to learn how to touch a patient so he feels comforted instead of annoyed. Some patients dislike being touched, especially when the meaning of the touch is unknown or misunderstood. That's why you should ask for permission before offering a touch. You could simply ask, "Would you mind?" or "Could you use . . . ?"

Sometimes, it helps to say something kind while touching a patient. For example, you might clasp a patient's hand to reassure him and then smile and say, "I know what you're going through is difficult. I'm here to help if you have any questions or concerns." This lets the patient know that your touch is a friendly gesture and not meant to threaten or harm him in any way.

Look for the Signs

It's also a good idea to observe a patient's overall body language when considering whether to use touch. Ask yourself:

- Does this patient look nervous or angry?
- Would a touch calm this patient or threaten her personal boundaries?

Go with your instincts. Some patients feel more comfortable when they are reassured verbally. Some patients respond to both talk and touch. Keep in mind that every patient is different and will require a different type of care from you.

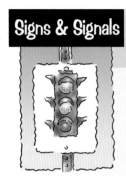

Signs & Signals

CULTURAL DIFFERENCES CONCERNING TOUCH

When using touch as a communication tool, it's important to be aware of cultural differences. For example, in certain cultures, touch is reserved for intimate acquaintances and family members only. (You'll learn more about cultural differences in Chapter 5.)

Patients who are uncomfortable with touch because of cultural or religious reasons might receive it negatively. Instead of communicating reassurance, a pat on the back might be perceived as an invasion of someone's personal space.

However, remember that each patient is unique, regardless of cultural background. The best approach is to observe each patient's body language to determine whether touch would be appropriate in a given situation.

Laughter as Medicine

There is some truth to the old saying "Laughter is the best medicine." Laughing increases blood flow and improves immune system function. It makes sense then that medical professionals would use humor to help patients feel comfortable. If patients see that you can laugh at yourself and see the humor in a situation, they will feel more comfortable opening up to you.

However, it's important for your humor to be tasteful and appropriate. Making a joke about someone's race or ethnicity, sexual orientation, gender, religion, or mental or physical capacity is never acceptable. It's also inappropriate to make jokes about a patient's condition or health problems. And it's a good idea to avoid sensitive areas and topics, such as politics, which may make a patient feel stressed or angry. If used correctly, however, humor can be a powerful therapeutic tool when communicating with patients.

> Tap into a patient's "funny bone" with humor.

Communicating with Coworkers

We've talked a lot about patient communication. It's important to keep in mind that as a medical assistant, you'll also be communicating with your coworkers. Communicating with coworkers is an active process. The quality of the communication depends on how well both parties:

- listen to one another
- ask questions
- share their ideas with one another

You are sharing the same space, so it's important to be courteous and respectful to your coworkers. You may not enjoy spending time with a coworker on a personal level, but as a professional, you should learn to put that aside and focus on coming together to provide good patient care.

WORKING WITH YOUR PEERS

Working with your peers can be a positive and rewarding experience. When you work with your peers, you learn to:

- use your communication skills effectively
- work as a team to accomplish a shared goal

Working with your peers demands focus and integrity on your part. You need to keep in mind that the job you're doing always comes first.

Communication with coworkers should remain professional. Discussion of topics that are not work related should be kept to a minimum or reserved for breaks only. It's not appropriate to discuss your personal problems in front of patients. Laughing, excessive or loud talking, and high-pitched voices can present an unprofessional image as well.

You can encourage communication among your peers by joining a local professional organization. By joining a group, you can learn more about your profession and meet others with similar interests and goals. Involvement in local community organizations can also help generate interest in medical assisting as a profession.

The Right Attitude

Has anyone ever told you to "stay positive"? It may sound easy to do, but stress can build up over time and result in a negative **attitude.** Your attitude is simply your state of mind or how you're feeling about something. Your attitude, whether positive or negative, affects your communication with others. In the medical office, not only does a negative attitude create an unpleasant work environment, it can disrupt the teamwork necessary to providing excellent patient care! Therefore, it's important to keep a positive attitude when communicating with coworkers.

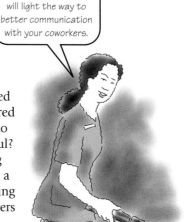

A positive attitude will light the way to better communication with your coworkers.

Think about the difference between being asked politely to perform a certain task and being ordered rudely to do the same task. Wouldn't you prefer to work with someone who was polite and respectful? Keeping a positive attitude while communicating with coworkers shows courtesy and respect. Also, a positive attitude can be contagious! By maintaining a positive attitude, you'll be helping your coworkers communicate well and work together as a team.

Although you may have bad days now and then, learn to leave your personal problems at the door when you arrive at work. Always enter the medical office with a positive professional attitude. Your attitude and behavior should present a positive image to patients and staff members alike.

Can't We All Just Get Along?

Consider the following scenario. Two friends are traveling to a party and get lost on a deserted road. They pull out their map. It's full of twists and turns, and neither person is quite sure which road to take. "It's this way," one says. "No, we have to go that way," says the other. The friends begin arguing. Neither wants to listen to the other. It grows dark, and they miss the party. They realize how foolish they were; they wasted their time and didn't get anywhere.

Does this scenario sound familiar? Getting along with coworkers can present a similar challenge. Your destination is the same, but you might have different ideas about the best way to get there. You have to work together to provide the best care possible to patients. This means using good communication skills so neither coworker is left stranded in the dark.

Patient Safety Comes First

You may come across a situation that requires you to speak to your supervisor about a coworker's actions. If this happens, follow these guidelines.

- Keep the information confidential. Don't gossip about the situation with patients or other coworkers.

Signs & Signals   DEALING WITH CONFLICTS

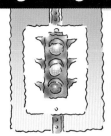

Conflicts will happen, but there are ways of dealing with them. Here's a list of do's and don'ts when dealing with conflicts.

- Stay calm; maintain a professional attitude.
- Put things in perspective. Ask yourself, "Will this really matter a day from now?"
- Explain what you did and why you did it.
- Use good verbal and nonverbal communication skills.
- Listen; every story has two sides.
- Ask questions if you don't understand something.
- Don't argue in front of patients, as this can upset them and present the staff as unprofessional and unapproachable.

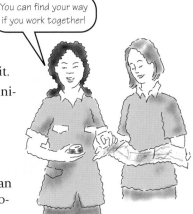

You can find your way if you work together!

- When you notify an appropriate supervisor, present facts as accurately and honestly as possible. Exaggerating or hiding information is not acceptable and may even cause you to lose your job.

Remember that you have a responsibility to your patients to provide the best care possible. If you see a coworker doing something that may harm a patient, tell a supervisor immediately. Maintaining patient safety is more important than protecting a coworker from disciplinary action.

Keep It Professional

As a medical assistant, it will be your job to communicate with many different personalities from a variety of backgrounds throughout the day. It's important to show the same level of courtesy to all coworkers. You may disagree with the private choices a coworker makes, but as a medical professional, your personal feelings should never affect your behavior toward him. Every coworker is an equally important part of the medical team and should be treated with respect.

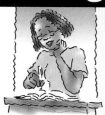

Travelog

COMMUNICATING TO RESOLVE CONFLICTS

What a week! Our first group project was due yesterday—I thought my group would never make it. A few students in the group didn't get along from the start. One person, Janice, took charge and began assigning parts of the project to each person. She just started ordering people around—I have to admit, it made me a little angry. A few students in the group started arguing with her. Pretty soon, they were almost shouting, and we got kicked out of the campus library!

At least one of the students in our group stayed calm and handled things well. After we left the library, we went outside and he suggested that we discuss who should complete certain parts of the project. Each person had a chance to speak to the group—and because no one was shouting, we could actually listen this time. Janice apologized for taking over. She explained that she was just worried about her grade and that she really wanted the project to go well. Everyone understood that—it's our first big project and we're all a little nervous. After we listened to each other, we were more comfortable working together. Each group member had something valuable to add—whether it was a research tip, a creative idea, or information we could use for the project. Once we learned how to communicate, we actually made a pretty good team!

COMMUNICATING WITH PHYSICIANS

The physician will depend on you to relay important information to patients in a timely manner. As a medical assistant, you'll be asked to keep the office running smoothly and efficiently. Nobody is perfect; miscommunications can happen. Remember, though, that you are a medical professional and your communication with the physician should reflect that.

R-E-S-P-E-C-T

When talking with the physician, always be courteous and respectful. You should address the physician by his appropriate title and last name unless otherwise specified. There's no need to feel intimidated when speaking to the physician. Speak slowly and confidently, and you'll develop a professional rapport with him.

The Right Words to Say

When relaying information about patients, never use inappropriate or slang terms. Instead, try to use correct medical terminology. If you don't know the correct terminology, describe the patient's condition to the physician. For example, when telling the physician about a patient who is experiencing dizziness and shortness of breath, say, "Ms. Estevez is complaining of dizziness and shortness of breath." A slang expression, such as "Her head is spinning," is inappropriate in the medical office.

Also, remember that the physician can help you if you don't understand something. If you need to clarify the physician's instructions, ask! It's better to ask than to assume you know the answer and make a mistake. Just remember to be respectful and to speak in a professional manner when asking the physician for help.

> Tell the physician that the patient is feeling dizzy instead of saying, "Her head is spinning."

Is It Appropriate?

Keep in mind that there is a time and a place for everything. A physician might enjoy discussing sports or telling jokes, but it's inappropriate to speak about these topics in front of patients and their family members. Professionalism doesn't mean you should be cold or unfriendly. Just remember to make sure the topics you're discussing are appropriate to the situation.

It's important to stick to appropriate conversation topics not just in the examination rooms, but whenever patients or their family members are in hearing distance. For example, if the waiting room is open to the receptionist's area, be aware of the volume and the tone of your voice. Always think about what you're saying and who is in hearing distance.

Using Communications Equipment

Have you ever been a passenger with a bad driver at the wheel? The driver just can't seem to stay in one lane, never uses a turn signal, or never learns to brake in time. At the end of the ride, you're a nervous wreck. You wonder how such a poor driver ever acquired a driver's license, and you wish someone would just take away the keys!

Using office equipment is a lot like driving—if you don't know how to operate the equipment properly, you might cause a problem for someone else. However, you'll have the respect of

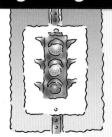

Signs & Signals   COMPLYING WITH HIPAA RULES

As you learned in Chapter 1, a federal law, HIPAA, was passed in 1996 to safeguard patient confidentiality. Compliance with HIPAA means that the medical office protects a patient's privacy and confidentiality at all times. Here are some tips to help you abide by HIPAA rules when you're communicating with other people in the medical office.

- Never share a patient's private medical information, either verbally or in writing, with anyone other than the patient unless you have the patient's permission to do so. (There are some exceptions to this rule which will be discussed later in this book.)

- When you must discuss private health information with a patient, find an office, an empty examination room, or another private area where other patients can't hear you.

- Never give out a patient's health information to someone other than the patient over the phone, even if that person claims to have the patient's permission.

- When communicating with patients over the phone, be aware of the volume of your voice when other people are within hearing distance.

- Never leave written documents containing a patients' private health information in an area where other patients can view it.

patients and other staff members if you know how to communicate effectively using:

- the phone
- the teletypewriter (TTY) device
- the fax machine
- e-mail

As a medical professional, you must learn to use communications equipment to communicate well with others.

TELEPHONES

The telephone is one of the most important devices you'll use in a medical office. You'll use the telephone to contact the medical community, including hospitals, pharmacies, and other physicians. The telephone also gives the patient access to immediate medical care and information. Patients will call to:

- schedule appointments
- report progress
- refill prescriptions
- obtain test results
- seek medical advice
- ask questions about their medical bills

As a medical assistant, it will be your job to communicate a positive image of the medical office without the help of non-verbal clues, like facial expressions and gestures. Therefore, you must use the tone and quality of your voice to send a message of genuine concern to patients. Also, because you can't see patients' body language when communicating over the phone, you may need to ask additional questions. By being courteous, paying attention to your expression, and listening actively, you'll communicate effectively and inspire confidence.

Taking Phone Messages

When taking phone messages for the physician or other coworkers, it's necessary to collect all the appropriate information from the caller. The minimum information needed for a phone message includes:

- the name of the caller
- the date and time of the call
- a phone number where the caller can be reached
- a brief description of the reason for the call
- the person for whom the message is intended

The recipient of the message will need this information so that he may return the call later. Callback times can vary from office to office. Some physicians return all calls at the end of the day, and others return calls randomly throughout the day. Be familiar with your office's policy so that you can tell the caller when to expect a return call.

PHONE MESSAGE

(1) Date: _1/27/2009_   Time: _2:30 P.M._
(2) For: _Dr. Parker_
(3) From: _Rosa Benitez_
(4) Phone: _(555) 234-5678_

(5) Message: _Mrs. Benitez would like to know if her test_
results are back.

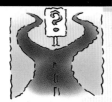

Fork in the Road

KEY INFORMATION

The following is a phone conversation between a medical assistant and a patient. Note key information communicated during the conversation and then write a phone message for the appropriate office staff member. Be sure to include the five necessary elements in your phone message.

Medical assistant: Good morning, Minneapolis Medical Associates. This is Keisha speaking. How may I help you?

Patient: Yes, hello, I'd like to speak with Dr. Harrington please.

Medical assistant: I'm sorry, Dr. Harrington is with a patient at the moment. May I take a message and have her call you back?

Patient: Sure, that would be fine. My name is Elizabeth Green and I'm calling to request a referral to see my dermatologist, Dr. Lopez.

Medical assistant: Have you already scheduled an appointment with Dr. Lopez?

Patient: Yes, my appointment is scheduled for tomorrow, May sixth.

Medical assistant: I'll be sure to let Dr. Harrington know. Should I have her call you at home?

Patient: Actually, I can be reached at work. My phone number is 333-456-0000, extension 4410.

Medical assistant: Thank you, Ms. Green. Dr. Harrington should be able to return your call in a half-hour, at ten o'clock.

Patient: That will be fine. Thanks!

PHONE MESSAGE

(1) Date: _____ Time: _____
(2) For: _____
(3) From: _____
(4) Phone: _____

(5) Message: _____
_____
_____
_____
_____

Perfecting Phone Manners

Showing **courtesy** means being polite and respectful. When speaking over the phone:

- Use the manners that you would use in person, such as saying "please" and "thank you."
- Address the caller by title and last name. For example, if Dr. Michelle Linh calls, never refer to her by her first name only.
- Treat each caller with the same level of courtesy.

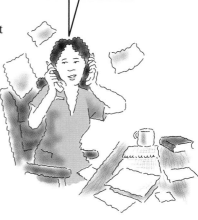

No matter how busy you are, you should always be polite and professional when answering the office phone. And remember to smile!

You'll receive many phone calls throughout the day that will interrupt your work. However, you shouldn't convey your irritation or impatience over the phone. Remember that you're there to help patients. Never answer a phone call by putting the caller on hold. If you're in the middle of a task, ask the caller if he would mind holding. Wait for a reply before you place the caller on hold. If you place a caller on hold, apologize for the delay when you pick up the phone again.

Express Yourself

Can you express a professional attitude even if a patient can't see you? Absolutely! When you talk on the phone, your expression is in the tone, pitch, and quality of your voice. The following are some tips to use when communicating on the phone.

- Sit up straight. Good posture has a positive effect on your health and even your attitude.
- Gather and organize your thoughts. If you don't understand what you're trying to say, neither will the patient.
- Speak clearly. A patient may become frustrated and impatient if he can't understand what you're saying.
- Speak slowly and confidently.
- Speak in a pleasant tone of voice. Remember that on the phone the sound of your voice helps you express yourself.

If a patient says he can't hear you, speak up. Just remember that when you're discussing a patient's health care concerns, the information is confidential. Always be aware of who is in hearing distance when speaking to a patient on the phone.

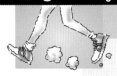

HELPING PATIENTS IN THE OFFICE AND OVER THE PHONE

How can you help patients in the office if you're already speaking to a caller on the phone?

At busy times, you may have to answer phone calls as well as communicate with patients face to face. Use your best judgment when handling both tasks.

- If you are talking to a patient or medical professional on the phone and a patient approaches your work area, acknowledge that person's presence and motion that you'll be with him just as soon as you can. Don't ignore him.

- If you know a call is going to be lengthy, ask the caller if she would mind holding. Then, address the needs of the patient in the office before returning to the call.

- Maintain patient confidentiality at all times. Avoid discussing private medical information with a caller if a patient in the office is standing nearby waiting to be helped.

- Remember that it's just as important to conduct yourself in a professional manner over the telephone as it is when communicating face to face.

Use Those Active Listening Skills

When you greet a patient over the phone, speak with enthusiasm. If a patient is receiving bad news, express your concern and empathy. Your voice should correspond to the situation. You must listen actively to understand how a patient is feeling and adjust the tone of your voice to meet the needs of the patient.

Listening actively also means that all your attention is on the conversation. You should ignore outside distractions and focus on what the person is saying. Avoid interrupting the speaker. Allow the speaker to complete her thought before asking questions or giving a response.

If you don't understand something that was said, ask for clarification. Verify that you've understood what was said by repeating the message. If the speaker asks you to do something, such as relay information to the physician or contact an insurance company, assure the speaker that you'll take the necessary actions.

Remember that you won't be able to use a speaker's nonverbal clues when communicating over the phone. Therefore, you'll have to listen twice as hard to ensure that both you and the speaker are understood.

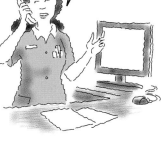

I'm sorry, it sounded like you said you've been feeling mnuph and rrpth. Could you please repeat that?

TELETYPEWRITER (TTY) DEVICES

Patients who have hearing or speech impairments often require special equipment to communicate using the phone. Teletypewriter (TTY) devices (also called text phones or telecommunication devices for the deaf) enable these patients to communicate through typed messages. Most medical offices have a TTY device or access to one. As a medical assistant, you should learn how to use this device to communicate with special-needs patients.

Answering Calls

When answering a TTY call:

1. When you answer the phone and hear silence or a beeping sound, recognize that you may be receiving a TTY call.
2. Place the receiver in the TTY's acoustic coupler.
3. Turn the TTY's on/off switch to the ON position.
4. Type a short greeting, being sure to include your name and the name of the medical office. End your greeting with the abbreviation GA (which means "go ahead").

Placing Calls

When placing a TTY call:

1. Place the phone receiver in the acoustic coupler.
2. Turn the TTY's on/off switch to the ON position.
3. Dial the phone number and pay attention to the TTY's red signal lights. When the phone is ringing, the light will blink slowly. Fast blinking flashes, on the other hand, indicate that the line is busy.
4. Allow the phone to ring at least seven times to give the person enough time to respond to the call.
5. The person answering the call will then type a short greeting, followed by the abbreviation GA. After reading the greeting, type your response, being sure to include your name and the name of the medical office.

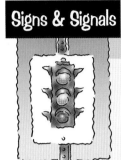

Signs & Signals

WHEN IT COUNTS THE MOST: EMERGENCY CALLS

While working in a medical office, you may receive a call that is a medical emergency. How do you know what constitutes an emergency? The following symptoms should be treated as emergencies:

- severe pain
- profuse bleeding
- respiratory distress
- chest pain
- loss of consciousness or changes in the level of consciousness
- severe vomiting or diarrhea
- temperature above 102 degrees F
- numbness
- vision changes

Keep in mind that this is an incomplete list. If you're ever unsure whether a particular symptom qualifies as an emergency, err on the side of caution and treat it as an emergency situation.

The following are some tips for handling emergency phone calls.

- Calm the caller by completely focusing on the call and listening attentively.
- Ask specific questions concerning the patient's condition. This will help determine whether the call is an emergency and how to handle it.
- Write down important information.
- If it's an emergency, immediately notify the physician or another qualified health care professional (such as the office nurse).
- Determine the patient's name, location, and phone number as quickly as possible in case the call becomes disconnected.
- The office should have a policy concerning how to handle emergencies after hours. Usually, the patient is directed to go to the nearest emergency room or call emergency services (911).

Signs & Signals

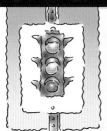

TTY CONVERSATION TIPS

Here are several tips to help you conduct successful TTY conversations.

- Use standard TTY abbreviations, such as GA ("go ahead"), HD ("hold"), Q (question mark), and SK ("stop keying" or "good-bye").
- Wait for the other person to type GA before typing your response.
- If you're unable to read a person's message, you may interrupt by typing a brief message, such as STOP HD CAN'T RD U or STOP PLS. Then, ask the person to retype the message.
- If you make a typing mistake, type XXX to indicate the error and then retype the word or phrase. Some TTY devices allow you to delete the error by using the back-space key.
- When you're ready to end the conversation, type GA OR SK ("go ahead or stop keying"). This gives the other person the option of continuing the conversation or hanging up.

TELECOMMUNICATIONS RELAY SERVICES

If your office is not equipped with a TTY device, you may communicate with deaf and hard-of-hearing patients through telecommunications relay services (TRS). These services are required by the federal government and must be available 24 hours a day.

Here's how TRS works:

1. The TTY user contacts a TRS provider (also called a "relay center").
2. A communications assistant (CA) who works for the TRS provider then places a call to the voice user.
3. The TTY user types messages to the CA, who reads the messages aloud to the voice user.
4. The voice user responds verbally to the CA, who types the messages for the TTY user.

TRS providers are the "go-betweens" who help TTY users communicate with people who don't have access to TTY devices. Voice users can also place calls to people who are deaf or hard of hearing by contacting a TRS provider.

FAX MACHINES

Facsimile, or fax, machines allow the medical office to send and receive printed documents over a phone line. Fax machines offer a convenient and affordable way to transmit materials such as patient records, orders, prescriptions, test results, and other items.

Playing by the Rules

HIPAA rules determine how protected health information is handled in the medical office. According to HIPAA, medical professionals may use a fax machine to send private patient information. However, certain guidelines must be followed.

- Only use a fax machine that is located in a private area of the office, away from patient foot traffic. Some medical offices may have two fax machines: one for general office use and another for faxing protected health information.

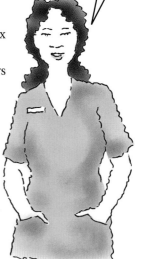

Make sure the right person is there to receive your fax—call ahead before sending confidential information.

- Always include a cover sheet with a confidentiality statement. (See the sample cover sheet on page 71.)
- Make sure the recipient is there to receive the fax and pick it up immediately.
- Verify the correct fax number or use fax numbers that are preprogrammed into the fax machine.
- If a fax is accidentally sent to the wrong recipient, make sure it's destroyed. Document the error according to office policy and take steps to prevent the error from happening again.
- Save fax transmittal confirmations for future verification.
- When confidential information is faxed to your office, make sure a staff member who is authorized to view the information retrieves the fax immediately.

Anatomy of a Cover Sheet

It's important to include a cover sheet when faxing confidential documents. The cover sheet should include the following information:

- name, address, telephone, and fax number of the physician's office

- name of the person intended to receive the fax
- number of pages being sent, including the cover sheet
- date the fax was sent
- confidentiality statement

Bay City Family Practice
123 Main Street
Anytown, USA 0000
(555) 555-5555
(555) 555-1234

facsimile transmittal

To: Dr. Alek Oblimov, Cardiology Associates   Fax: (333) 555-3333

From: Dr. Melissa Jones   Date: 8/10/2009

Re: Patient consult   Pages: 6

CC:

☐ Urgent   ☐ For Review   ☐ Please Comment   ☐ Please Reply   ☐ Please Recycle

Comments:

CONFIDENTIAL INFORMATION

The information contained in this message and any accompanying documents is private and confidential. This information is intended only for the eyes of the addressee. If you are not the intended recipient of this information, you are hereby notified that any disclosure, copying or distribution of this information is strictly prohibited. Please notify the sender immediately by telephone.

E-MAIL

Electronic mail, or e-mail, is an important form of communication within the health care system. E-mail promotes teamwork among staff and helps you provide efficient patient care. E-mail is also important because it provides written documentation of sent and received messages.

Keep Things Professional

When you send an e-mail, you are using written communication to convey a message to the receiver. You're also presenting an overall image of the medical office. If your e-mail is unprofessional, it will leave a negative impression on the person receiving it. The following are guidelines for composing and sending e-mails.

- Avoid using your personal e-mail account to send work-related messages. Likewise, avoid sending personal messages from your work e-mail address.

- When you're out of the office, always leave a message on your e-mail system letting others know that you're away and when you'll be back.

- Use professional language; avoid using slang or incorrect grammar. Also, avoid using emoticons (such as smiley faces) when sending work-related e-mails.

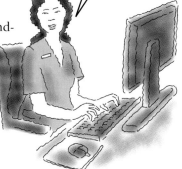

Like all written communication in the medical office, e-mails should always be professional.

- Keep messages brief and straightforward. Your e-mail should be no more than one screen page in length and should focus on one topic.

- Check your spelling and grammar before sending each e-mail.

- Use appropriate font size and style.

- Flag messages of high importance. This lets others know that the e-mail you sent requires an immediate response.

- Always complete the subject line. This gives the receiver an idea of what the message is regarding.

Respect Patients' Privacy

E-mail isn't guaranteed to provide patient confidentiality. However, there are a few things you can do to ensure that patients' privacy is respected. Here are some guidelines to follow when using e-mail.

- Open only your own e-mail messages unless otherwise instructed.

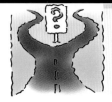

Fork in the Road   E-MAIL ETIQUETTE

Read the following e-mail from a medical assistant to a patient. There are a number of things wrong with this e-mail. First, list at least five elements in the e-mail that make it unprofessional. Then, rewrite the e-mail correctly.

To: Steve Warner <s_warner@email.com>
From: Carla Sanchez <i_love2shop@yahoo.com>
Date: 26 Feb 2009
Subject: [none]

Hey Steve,

We got your request to have your medical records transferred to Dr. Wen's office. No problem!!! I'll have those records sent over as soon as I finish my lunch. ☺

There will be a fee of $200 (JK, LOL). There's no fee for transferring your records to another physician.

Just let me know if you need anthing els!

Carla Sanchez, CMA

—
Family Medical Group
100 Medical Parkway, Suite 101
Anytown, USA 12345
Phone: (555) 123-1000
Fax: (555) 123-4567
E-mail Carla.Sanchez@medicalgroup.com

The information contained in this e-mail is confidential and intended for the sole use of the individual named above. If you are not the intended recipient, please delete this e-mail immediately.

- After reading an e-mail, delete it or save it in a folder.
- Be discreet. Avoid leaving private messages on the screen where others can read them. Only read confidential e-mails when other members of the staff are away from your immediate work area.
- Forward a patient's confidential e-mail only to the appropriate person, usually the physician or another office staff member. Don't discuss patients' e-mails outside the office.
- Activate the encryption feature for your e-mail account. Encryption scrambles the sent message so it can't be read until it reaches the recipient.
- Include a privacy statement (similar to the one described for a fax) on all outgoing messages.

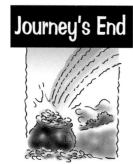

Journey's End

- Proper and effective communication skills are an important part of your interactions with patients and coworkers. Good communication skills put people at ease, send a positive message, and let others know that you care and want to help.

- Nonverbal communication uses facial expressions, gestures, and body language to convey messages. Paying attention to body language will help you know your patient's needs and respond accordingly.

- Active listening means you are mentally and physically engaged with what the other person is communicating to you.

- Therapeutic communication involves touching patients, allowing silences, and using humor to provide effective patient care.

- Therapeutic communication is important because it allows you to connect with the patient on a more personal level for better care and treatment.

- A successful medical team uses good communication skills to work together and resolve conflicts; working as a team also helps maintain a professional and courteous work environment.

- Teamwork is an important part of the health care setting. Coworkers must work together to complete tasks and provide high-quality patient care. Everyone should be focused on the same goal—professional patient care.

- Use office communications equipment effectively by following office procedures, adhering to HIPAA confidentiality rules, and presenting a professional image.

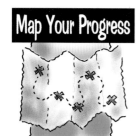

Map Your Progress

Answer the following multiple-choice questions.

1. Which of the following is NOT a form of nonverbal communication?
   a. smiling at a patient
   b. laughing at a joke
   c. saying, "I'm sorry"
   d. pointing your body toward a speaker

2. Which of the following is NOT a form of *kinesics*?
   a. eye movements
   b. nonlanguage sounds
   c. gestures
   d. facial expressions

3. What does *proxemics* refer to?

    a. a type of therapeutic touch used by medical professionals
    b. the type of communication that most people prefer
    c. the degree of physical closeness tolerated by humans
    d. the amount of emotional support a person requires

4. *Reflecting* is:
    a. restating what you have heard, using your own words.
    b. repeating what the patient said, using open-ended phrases or questions.
    c. asking the "what," "when," and "how" questions.
    d. reviewing what the patient has told you.

5. Touch can communicate:
    a. friendliness.
    b. concern.
    c. hostility.
    d. all of the above

6. If you're providing information to a physician and you don't know the correct medical terminology to use, what should you do?
    a. Describe the patient's condition to the physician.
    b. Find the answer in a medical textbook.
    c. Walk away.
    d. Call 911.

7. How can you safeguard a patient's confidentiality?
    a. Discuss the patient's health information with a trusted coworker.
    b. Discuss the patient's health information with her family.
    c. Leave the patient's health documents unattended.
    d. Take the patient to a private room before discussing health information.

8. Which of the following should you include in a phone message?
    a. what you were doing prior to receiving the call
    b. the caller's location
    c. date and time the call was received
    d. the caller's tone of voice

9. Which of the following signifies an emergency call?
    a. a persistent cough
    b. profuse bleeding
    c. a stomachache
    d. joint swelling

10. A TTY device can help you communicate over the phone with patients who are:
    a. hearing or speech impaired.
    b. bilingual.
    c. sight impaired.
    d. physically impaired.

Chapter 3

SERVICE WITH A SMILE

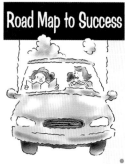

Road Map to Success

- Define customer service, including its relationship to professionalism

- Identify the customer in a heath care setting, and explain how to determine his needs

- Explain the importance of good customer service

- Describe how to make a good first impression

- Explain how a positive attitude can lead to patient trust and prevent conflict

- Describe proper waiting room management techniques

- Describe how to effectively manage challenging patients

- Summarize how your customer service skills can affect the entire health care facility

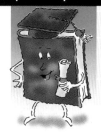

Chapter Competencies

- Project a positive attitude (ABHES 1.a.)

- Be courteous and diplomatic (ABHES 1.h.)

- Be impartial and show empathy when dealing with patients (ABHES 2.b.)

- Explain general office policies (CAAHEP 3.c.3.a.)

What exactly is customer service? What does it have to do with the medical office? This chapter answers these questions and more. In this chapter, you'll learn how to make a good first impression, why maintaining a positive attitude is important, and how to handle difficult situations that can occur in the medical office. You'll discover what goes into good customer service and how it all relates to your journey toward professionalism.

The Art of Customer Service

Just like the many other skills you're developing to become a successful medical assistant, customer service is a skill that requires practice. **Customer service** refers to the ways you help customers have a positive experience.

When you get a haircut, dine at a restaurant, or buy furniture, you're receiving a particular service. The people providing the service are there to help you and meet your consumer needs. But what is customer service, and why is it important to know about it as a medical assistant?

Good customer service includes the following:

- being able to identify and help meet customers' needs
- approaching difficult situations with a positive attitude
- showing courtesy at all times
- being competent and resourceful

WHO ARE YOUR "CUSTOMERS" IN A MEDICAL FACILITY?

In a medical facility, your "customers" are the patients, and customer service is the quality of care you provide to them. These customers are seeking high-quality care and attentiveness to their health concerns. As a medical assistant, the service you'll provide to each patient will involve making sure her experience with the medical office is a positive one. This may be as simple as greeting a patient warmly when she comes through the door, handling her insurance billing efficiently, or following proper procedures when conducting a patient interview or taking vital sign measurements.

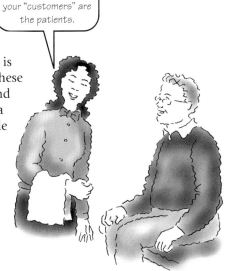

In the medical office, your "customers" are the patients.

WHY IS CUSTOMER SERVICE IMPORTANT?

So why is customer service important in the medical office? One reason is that the medical office is a business. A business can be successful only if customers keep returning. If patients are satisfied with the level of customer service they receive, they're more likely to return to the office. Patients who have unpleasant experiences with a particular medical office, however, may decide to change physicians.

Customer service is also important because it's an aspect of professionalism. A professional learns to treat his customers well because he cares about their well-being. He attends to their needs and has their best interests at heart. The medical profession is all about caring for others, so practicing good customer service is a natural extension of this principle.

There is also a legal reason why customer service is so important in health care. Patients who have good relationships with their health care providers are less likely to sue if there's a medical problem or negative outcome as a result of treatment. By providing good customer service, you'll help develop a good rapport between patients, the physician, and other staff members.

Identifying Your Customers' Needs

Although every patient has a set of unique needs, there are similarities among those needs. For example, a child may want you to hold her hand through a procedure, but an adult may prefer a reassuring phrase. The need for care and attention is the same, though it is expressed in different ways.

The well-known psychologist Abraham Maslow created a hierarchy of basic needs that all human beings share. (See the illustration on page 79.) A hierarchy means that there are different levels, and each level builds upon the one below it. Lower-level needs, such as the needs for food and shelter, must be met before higher-level needs can be met. In Maslow's hierarchy of human needs, the needs at the bottom of the pyramid are the more basic needs. Once a person's most basic survival needs have been met, he can concentrate on other, more complex needs, such as feeling secure in the world or finding friends to spend time with. People's needs affect the ways in which they live their lives, the choices they make, and the things they seek from themselves and others.

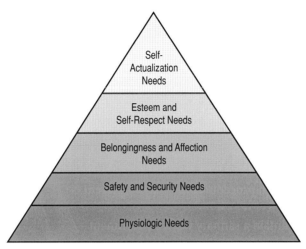

Maslow's hierarchy of human needs places the most basic needs at
the bottom of the pyramid and the higher-level needs at the top.

PHYSIOLOGIC NEEDS

Meeting physiologic needs is essential for survival. Physiologic
needs are the most basic needs, such as:

- oxygen
- water
- food
- shelter
- elimination (releasing waste products from the body, such
  as carbon dioxide, urine, and feces)
- rest and sleep
- sexuality (reproduction)

As a medical assistant, you probably won't be helping
patients meet these basic needs. However, nurses and physicians
often address these needs for patients in long-term care facilities
(such as nursing homes) and hospitals.

SAFETY AND SECURITY NEEDS

Once a person's physiologic needs have been met, the next level
in the hierarchy is safety and security needs. These needs are
both physical and emotional. Examples of safety and security
needs include the following:

- trusting others
- having no fear of physical or emotional harm; feeling
  unthreatened

- feeling certain that other needs will be met with the help of other people

As a medical assistant, you can help meet some of these needs by following policies and procedures that are designed to ensure patients' safety, such as the following.

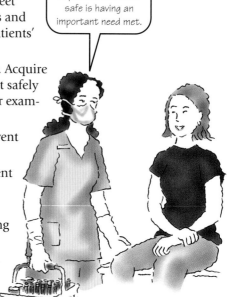

A patient who feels safe is having an important need met.

- Use all medical equipment properly. Acquire the necessary skills to use equipment safely before using it during a procedure or examination with a patient.
- Perform procedures correctly to prevent injury or infection.
- Maintain a sanitary work environment and practice good personal hygiene.
- Follow HIPAA rules, as well as your medical office's guidelines concerning patient privacy and confidentiality.
- Create a warm and friendly environment. Offer to assist the patient even if he doesn't look like he needs it.

LOVE AND BELONGING NEEDS

Love and belonging needs include feeling understood, accepted, and appreciated by others. People meet these needs in two ways:

- showing physical affection
- forming intimate relationships

Medical assistants help meet this need for patients by taking a professional interest in them as individuals, and not just as medical conditions or illnesses. Discuss with a patient how her health concerns are affecting her overall wellness. Ask her how she's feeling and if she needs help. Taking a sincere interest in a patient's well-being will let her know that you're invested in her health care at every step, from diagnosis to recovery. In fact, the information she shares with you could lead to even more effective care.

SELF-ESTEEM NEEDS

Self-esteem needs relate to a person's sense of self-worth. People who value themselves or feel valued by others have a healthy level of self-esteem.

In a health care setting, many things can affect patients' self-esteem, such as:

- having to disrobe for a physical examination
- having surgery that might change the person's physical appearance
- relearning basic motor coordination skills after an injury or accident
- fear of being judged by the medical staff

Medical assistants preserve patients' self-esteem by treating them with dignity, providing them with privacy, and assisting them with a caring and empathetic attitude.

SELF-ACTUALIZATION NEEDS

Self-actualization is the highest level in the hierarchy of needs. A patient who is self-actualized feels personal responsibility and control over his own life. This patient will be concerned with maintaining his own health and wellness and may even help others achieve wellness. However, self-actualization can be achieved only when all other needs have been met.

By making sure patients' other basic needs are met, you can help them reach self-actualization. But keep in mind that not all patients will reach this level. You can assist patients by helping them meet small, realistic goals. Examples of goals that you and the patient might set together include the following:

- walking around the house (as part of a physical therapy regimen)
- quitting smoking or stopping other addictions
- making a lifestyle change, such as complying with a special diet to control a medical condition

Making a Good First Impression

First impressions can last a long time. You have only one chance to make a first impression on patients. Because you'll most likely have contact with new patients before the physician does (whether it's over the phone, at the reception desk, or in an examination room), a patient's overall opinion of the medical office is often based on the impression you make.

Making a good first impression will let the patient know that you're a professional who cares about the quality of

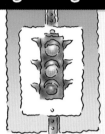

Signs & Signals

IDENTIFYING A PATIENT'S NEEDS

- Observe the patient's movements. For example, as you escort an older adult patient to an examination room, ask yourself, "Are his movements slow? Does he walk with a cane?" This patient may require assistance when walking. But be sure to ask him first if he'd like help. Don't make assumptions about a patient's level of need.

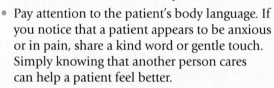

Sometimes, patients' needs are obvious. But other times, you may need to ask, "How may I help you?"

- Observe the patient's appearance. For example, if you notice that an older adult patient appears unkempt, you might determine that he needs more help at home.

- Pay attention to the patient's body language. If you notice that a patient appears to be anxious or in pain, share a kind word or gentle touch. Simply knowing that another person cares can help a patient feel better.

- Practice open and effective communication skills, including good listening, to help determine what's going on with a patient.

- There may be times when you're not sure what would improve the quality of care you're providing. In that situation, simply ask the patient, "How may I help you?"

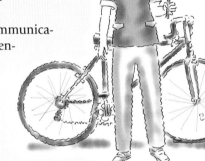

FLAT TIRE

health care you provide. Making a good impression depends on the following:

- having a professional manner and image
- using appropriate body language

MANNER AND IMAGE

Presenting a professional image to patients is the first step toward making a good first impression. Your appearance is the first thing a patient notices. Like it or not, people often make quick, unconscious judgments based on appearance. If a patient sees that you're well groomed and that your uniform is neat and clean, it's likely that her first impression will be a positive one. Maintaining a professional image shows that you take your work seriously. (See Chapter 5 for specific information about your physical appearance on the job.)

If looking the part is the first step toward making a good first impression, then acting the part is the next step. Show patients that you're committed to providing high-quality care by making sure your manner remains professional at all times. This may include handling difficult situations in a calm and professional way (which you'll read about later in this chapter). Or it may include simple acts such as smiling as you greet patients and speaking to patients in a pleasant and polite tone.

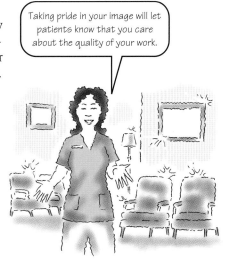

Taking pride in your image will let patients know that you care about the quality of your work.

If a patient can see right away that your manner and appearance are professional, then she'll be more likely to trust you to provide good care.

WHAT YOU SAY WITHOUT WORDS

As you learned in Chapter 2, body language includes the messages you send to others using facial expressions, gestures, and body movements. It's important to use body language that will make a good first impression on each patient. Use the following examples of good body language when interacting with patients.

- Make eye contact. Eye contact is a sign of respect that lets the patient know you're listening actively to what she's saying.
- Smile at the patient. Smiling can help relax an anxious patient. A smile can also communicate to patients that you're receptive and friendly.
- Position your body to face the patient. This movement implies that you're giving the patient your full attention.
- Use gestures that convey empathy and concern. For example, you might nod your head in understanding or touch the person's shoulder. Let the patient know that you're listening to what she has to say and are concerned for her welfare.

The Right Attitude Builds Trust

Another aspect of providing good customer service is having the right attitude. Your attitude reflects how you're feeling on the inside. It can be either positive or negative. Your attitude often affects what you say and how you act. In the medical office, a positive attitude can help you earn patients' trust and handle difficult situations in a professional way—both of which help meet patients' needs.

Be sure to leave any personal problems at the door upon entering the medical office. Everyone has bad days now and then, but your private life and your attitude concerning it shouldn't influence the quality of care you provide to patients. Keep in mind that discussing your personal problems with patients is unprofessional and may even make patients feel uncomfortable. However, if patients feel that your working attitude is stable and consistent, then they'll trust you to take good care of them.

Patients may have had unpleasant experiences with other medical offices in the past. Before a patient decides to place himself in your capable hands, he has to trust that he will be taken care of. Sometimes, it may take a while for the patient to develop this trust. You can encourage a patient to trust you by paying attention to the following trust-builders.

- Make the right first impression. A patient will form judgments based on his initial contact with you, and it can be hard to change his mind later on. So be friendly and prepared to meet new patients every day.

- Pay attention to your body language. Smiling when appropriate, making eye contact, and nodding your head are ways to let the patient know that you care and are listening to what he has to say.

- Be responsible. Follow through with the patient's questions and concerns. If you don't know the answer to something, then find out. A patient will trust you if he knows he can count on you as a reliable resource.

- Maintain patients' confidentiality. The patient will trust you if he knows his personal medical information will be kept private.

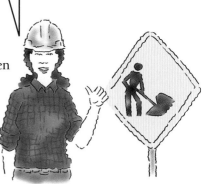

Trust is the foundation of a healthy physician-patient relationship. Do what you can to help build patients' trust!

Know Your Limits

Knowing your limits with patients also helps you handle difficult situations in a professional manner. To be a successful medical assistant, you'll need to establish limits by maintaining a professional distance with patients. Keep in mind that professional distance doesn't mean ignoring patients or being insensitive to their needs and concerns. It simply means that you should avoid becoming too personally involved in patients' lives.

When you're personally involved with a patient, it's more difficult to be objective and show impartiality, two elements that are necessary for providing high-quality patient care. By keeping a professional distance, you'll be able to handle difficult situations with the right attitude and a calm, professional manner.

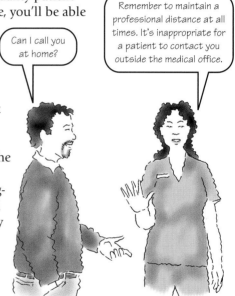

Can I call you at home?

Remember to maintain a professional distance at all times. It's inappropriate for a patient to contact you outside the medical office.

To keep a professional distance, avoid revealing intimate information about yourself. It's inappropriate to talk with patients about your marital problems, financial troubles, or family conflicts. Discussing these topics can shift the dynamics of the relationship to a more personal level. Likewise, avoid encouraging patients to share too much personal information with you. Listening politely to patients is acceptable, but patients shouldn't begin to depend on you to solve their personal problems or offer advice that is outside the scope of your professional practice.

Additionally, patients may misinterpret something you've said and become confused or offended. For example, you might attempt to console a patient who has recently been diagnosed with cancer by saying, "Don't worry. My grandmother had cancer, and she's fine now. You'll be fine, too." The patient might become offended and misinterpret this statement to mean that you don't think her diagnosis is a serious matter.

It's also incorrect to give patients false assurances. Only the physician can provide information about a patient's condition. If you tell a patient, "Don't worry, you'll be fine," but the physician tells her something different, she may become upset or angry. Although it's important to be friendly and understanding,

Travelog

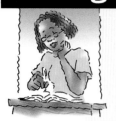

SETTING LIMITS WITH PATIENTS

Working part time at a physician's office has taught me a lot. Even though I've just been helping out with administrative tasks in the front office, it's given me a chance to see how the things I'm learning in school apply to an actual office environment. My coworkers have been really helpful, too—I've gotten a lot of good advice on how to deal with tough situations.

Just last month, one of my coworkers helped steer me in the right direction. One of the physician's patients, Mr. Saul, is an elderly man whose wife recently passed away. He just seemed lost without her—he no longer joked around with the office staff when he came in for his appointments, and it looked like he might have started losing weight, too.

I really wanted to do something that would help, so I asked my coworker if it would be OK to offer to do Mr. Saul's weekly grocery shopping or take a meal to him a few times a week. To my surprise, my coworker told me I definitely shouldn't do that! She said that, as health care professionals, we should avoid getting personally involved with patients because it can cloud our judgment. She explained that being objective is important because it helps us provide the best possible care to each patient.

So instead of offering to do Mr. Saul's grocery shopping, my coworker suggested that I do some research and find a few local organizations that might be able to help, such as support groups for grieving spouses or a local Meals on Wheels chapter. She also recommended that I mention my concerns to the physician so he could address any nutrition needs Mr. Saul may have.

I followed her advice, and I'm glad I did! Mr. Saul came in last week, and he looked a lot healthier. He still isn't quite back to joking with the office staff, but he seems to be doing much better.

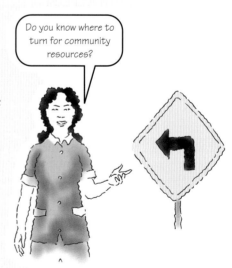

Do you know where to turn for community resources?

remember to keep a professional distance during all your interactions with patients.

Managing the Waiting Room

In the medical office, good customer service means providing a comfortable and safe waiting room environment. The waiting room gives patients their first glimpse of the medical office, so the atmosphere should be warm and welcoming.

As a medical assistant, you may be responsible for doing things such as making sure the waiting area remains clean and uncluttered or selecting appropriate reading materials. Sometimes, it also helps to sit in the waiting room for a bit to see it as patients see it. This can help you find ways of making the

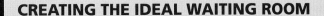

Road Rules CREATING THE IDEAL WAITING ROOM

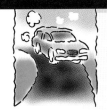

- Keep the waiting area clean and uncluttered. Chairs should be arranged to allow patients plenty of room to maneuver around one another.
- Make sure the waiting room is kept at a comfortable temperature.
- Control the noise level in the front office. If a television is present, set the volume to a reasonable level, or keep it turned off unless a patient requests to watch a television program.
- Make sure television programs are appropriate. Avoid selecting shows with violence, strong language, or sexual content. Posting a simple sign, such as, "Please see the receptionist for channel changes," prevents patients from choosing programs that may be inappropriate for the office.
- Set out patient education materials, such as brochures or pamphlets. Patients may take them home or read them while they wait, and they can feel comfortable learning about medical topics they might have otherwise been too uncomfortable to ask about.
- Provide a wide range of magazines and leisure reading material appropriate to the patients you treat. Make sure reading materials are up to date and in good condition.

waiting room more comfortable, such as rearranging furniture, organizing educational materials, and so forth.

Managing the waiting room also involves interacting with patients. In the following sections, you'll learn the proper way to greet patients when they come into the office, educate new patients about office policies, manage patients' waiting time, and end each patient's visit to the office.

GREETING PATIENTS

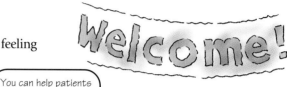

In our hectic, fast-paced world, feeling valued and appreciated can seem like a luxury. At times, it may seem as if no one has the time to say a simple "Hello. How are you today?" This is why greeting patients properly is so important—they should feel that you notice them, value their concerns, and truly want to help. If you take the time to greet patients as they enter the office, they may feel more relaxed and comfortable during their visits.

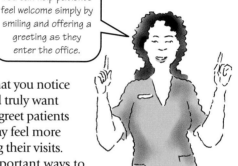

You can help patients feel welcome simply by smiling and offering a greeting as they enter the office.

The following are some important ways to make patients feel welcome.

- Greet patients personally and by name. For example, you might say, "Good morning, Mr. Raza."
- Smile when speaking with patients. Smiling conveys a friendly, positive attitude.
- Speak in a pleasant and cheerful tone of voice.
- Try to remember a personal fact about each patient. For example, if Mrs. Martinez loves taking her dog for walks, you might ask, "How is your cocker spaniel, Mrs. Martinez?"
- A patient may arrive when you're away from the reception desk. Be sure to scan the waiting room for new arrivals when you return and greet them warmly.

WELCOMING AND ORIENTING NEW PATIENTS

In managing the waiting area, you'll also encounter new patients. Patients who are new to the office must fill out a registration form. In most medical offices, patients complete these forms themselves and ask for help if questions arise. However, you may be asked to fill out a patient's registration form as you conduct the new patient interview. A registration form typically includes the following information about a patient:

- name
- address
- phone number
- health insurance information
- employer's name and address
- marital status
- emergency contact information
- Social Security number
- name of the referring physician (if referrals are required by the patient's insurance plan)

After registration, you'll *orient* the new patient to the office. You can do this by helping the patient become familiar with the office and its policies.

- Give the patient brochures and cards with the names of the physician and staff, office hours, and phone numbers.
- Explain any important office policies or procedures concerning billing, appointment cancellations, and parking.
- Point out the water fountain and restroom, but remind the patient to check with you before using the restroom to find out whether a urine specimen is needed.

You may also take the patient back to the examination room at the appropriate time. Your goal is to make the registration and orientation process as simple and smooth as possible.

MANAGING WAITING TIME

Aside from greeting each patient and helping new patients become familiar with the medical office, you may also be responsible for managing waiting time. Patients often must take time off from work and other responsibilities to visit the physician's office. They have a limited amount of time in their schedules and don't want to be kept waiting. Sometimes, even if you do everything right, delays can still occur. The physician may be running late one morning or a patient may need to come in for an emergency visit. So how do you manage waiting time for patients when things happen that are beyond your control? Here are a few helpful tips to keep in mind.

- Tell patients if the physician is running behind schedule. Patients will appreciate your honesty and can adjust their schedules accordingly.

- If you expect a patient's waiting time to be 30 minutes or more past her appointment time, offer her some choices. The patient may choose to leave and come back later in the day or reschedule the appointment for another time.

- Be firm, but polite. Apologize to patients for the inconvenience. Being courteous shows that you care.

SEEING PATIENTS OUT

Just as it's important to greet patients as they enter the office, it's also essential to see patients out properly at the end of each visit.

After the physician has completed a patient's examination, the patient will be asked to dress and wait for her discharge information. Depending on office policy, you may be assigned the task of educating the patient about the physician's instructions or providing the patient with information about prescribed medications. Ensure that the patient understands the instructions, and

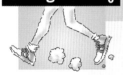

Running Smoothly

WAITING WOES

What if patients become upset about the wait?

It's been a busy morning, and the physician is running behind schedule. It's 11:00 A.M., and the physician is just now seeing the patient who had a 10:15 appointment. There are three patients in the waiting room, and they are starting to complain about the long wait. One patient approaches the reception desk and tells you that he has to be across town in 45 minutes and can't possibly wait any longer to see the physician. How can you manage the waiting time in a way that will be satisfactory for all three patients?

When managing waiting time for several patients, follow these two steps.

- First, be honest about the wait. Speak with each patient individually to let him know how much longer the wait will be.

- Second, if you expect the wait to be longer than 30 minutes or more past each patient's scheduled appointment time, offer several choices. Patients may choose to wait for the physician, leave and return to the office later in the day, or reschedule their appointments for a later date.

address any questions the patient has before leaving the examination room to ensure patient privacy. Also, be sure to provide the patient with any appropriate pamphlets or written instructions.

You will then escort the patient to the front desk, where the receptionist will collect any necessary fees or copayment. If the physician has requested a follow-up visit, you may be responsible for scheduling the appointment. It's helpful to give each patient an appointment reminder card to take home.

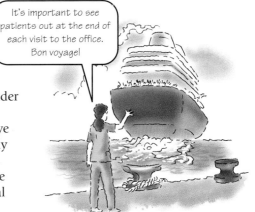

It's important to see patients out at the end of each visit to the office. Bon voyage!

Finally, remember to say good-bye to the patient in a warm and friendly manner. As patients leave the office, you want them to feel that they have been well cared for by a professional and courteous staff.

The Customer Is King (or Queen)

A large part of customer service involves going the extra mile to keep the customer happy. In the medical office, you can provide good customer service by making an effort to be courteous and tactful. Handling patients with courtesy and tact can help:

- increase your awareness of patients' needs
- prevent potential conflicts or misunderstandings

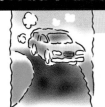

Road Rules

PATIENT VISITS: FROM GREETING TO GOOD-BYE

- Smile and greet patients warmly. If you seem relaxed and comfortable, you will help patients feel the same.
- When meeting new patients, have them fill out the proper registration forms or complete the forms with them during the initial interview.
- Keep patients informed about waiting time and offer choices if you expect the wait to be longer than 30 minutes.
- At the end of each visit, answer any questions patients may have, and don't forget to say good-bye when they leave.

- build strong rapport and trust between patients and medical office staff

COURTESY

When you show courtesy to others, you treat them with respect. As a medical assistant, you can show courtesy to patients by being sensitive to their needs and feelings. You can also display courtesy by using good manners and maintaining a positive attitude.

But why is courtesy so important? Showing all patients the same respect and courtesy helps you earn patients' trust. Being courteous also puts patients at ease. Patients who feel relaxed and comfortable are more likely to be open about their health concerns, which allows you to help the physician provide the best possible care. And when patients' health care needs are met, they become satisfied customers.

To show courtesy to patients, follow these tips.

- Remember to include polite phrases such as "please," "thank you," and "excuse me," in all interactions with patients.

- Use terms patients can understand (as opposed to medical jargon) but avoid "talking down" or being condescending to patients. For example, calling patients "honey" or "sweetie" is inappropriate.

- Address people as they prefer to be addressed. When you're unsure, be cautious and use the proper title and last name, such as "Mr. Yang" or "Ms. Monroe."

DIPLOMACY

Diplomacy is the ability to handle people with graciousness and tact. A diplomatic person sees all sides of a situation and tries to find a balance or compromise that will satisfy everyone involved. Diplomacy is used in difficult situations that can occur in the medical office, such as:

- when a patient is irritable about a prolonged waiting time

- when a patient is ill or in pain and wants to see the physician immediately

- when an unauthorized person requests confidential patient information

Occasionally, someone may make a request that you can't grant. For example, patients may be curious about other patients, or family members may ask what the physician said to the patient. In these situations, a polite refusal is appropriate. A diplomatic response might be a simple explanation that it's against office policy to give out confidential patient information.

At other times, it may be necessary to provide several options or choices. If a patient becomes irritable or confrontational, you must exercise self-control and use an understanding, but firm, approach. As you learned earlier in this chapter, never argue with a patient. Instead, try to calm the patient and communicate your desire to help.

A diplomatic approach to providing customer service keeps you in control of yourself and shows professionalism.

FOCUS ON PROVIDING GOOD PATIENT CARE

One of the most important ways you can provide good customer service and show professionalism is by providing high-quality care, such as:

- being resourceful
- being impartial
- showing compassion and empathy
- making sure patients are comfortable
- being sensitive to patients' vulnerabilities

Be Resourceful

It's important to place patients' interests first. Always take the time to address patients' concerns and answer their questions. And if you don't know the answer to a question, find the appropriate person in the office who can address the patient's needs. The patient may need to talk to the office manager about insur-

Fork in the Road   **MAINTAINING DIPLOMACY**

Read the following scenario about a difficult situation that might occur in the medical office. In two to three sentences, write what you would say in response to the patient. Remember to use those diplomacy skills!

A patient's mother demands to see her son's medical records, but the patient is no longer a minor. You ask the patient if his mother may see them, but he refuses.

ance or billing problems, or to the physician about medical concerns that you can't address.

Sometimes, providing good customer service means going the extra mile. Being resourceful and seeking out accurate information is the mark of a true professional. Impress patients with good follow-through by being resourceful and making sure all their questions have been answered.

> Let patients know that they're number one—place patients' needs first!

Be Impartial

You may find that some patients are more pleasant to interact with than others. But you must treat all patients with the same level of care and courtesy. Be sensitive to each patient's needs, but remember that remaining professional is the name of the game. Being impartial requires you to keep a healthy professional distance and treat all patients equally.

Show Compassion and Empathy

Having compassion means you understand someone else's pain and feel compelled to do something about it. You learned about empathy in Chapter 2. Empathy is compassion in action. When you respond empathetically to someone, you try to put yourself in that person's shoes. You make an effort to understand not only *how* that person is feeling, but also *why* she feels that way. By demonstrating empathy and compassion in the medical office, you show each patient that she is important and that you care about her health needs.

There are several ways to show compassion and empathy in your duties as a medical assistant. One is by trying to help patients feel more comfortable before and during medical procedures. Another way to show compassion and empathy is by being sensitive to patient vulnerability.

Patient Comfort Is Key

By thinking about how you would like to be treated as a patient, you can show empathy in the way you perform your daily tasks in the medical office. For example, before conducting a procedure, you can help a patient feel more comfortable by letting him know what is going to happen. If you need to draw a blood specimen and the patient appears nervous, explain exactly what you're going to do before you begin. You might begin by saying, "First, I'm going to apply the tourniquet to your arm." Allow the patient to ask any questions before you begin. Then, talk the patient through each step as you complete it. Let the patient know when the procedure is almost over, especially if the patient seems to be experiencing pain or discomfort.

When assisting the physician with procedures, try to make the patient feel as comfortable as possible. Be aware of room temperature, give the patient a blanket or pillow to prop up a part of the body, or do whatever else might help a patient feel more comfortable. For example, you might offer to hold a young patient's hand if the child appears nervous about the procedure. As long as your actions don't interfere with the patient's recovery or healing, seeking to increase patient comfort is an excellent way to provide good customer service.

It's important to be able to "read" the patient to determine how detailed your explanation of the procedure should be. For a more knowledgeable patient, a less detailed explanation may be fine.

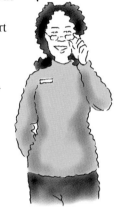

Being Sensitive to Patient Vulnerability

Another way to show empathy and compassion is to be sensitive to patient vulnerability. Situations that can lead patients to feel vulnerable include the following:

- disrobing before examinations or procedures
- wearing a dressing gown
- revealing personal sexual history or other medical information
- reacting negatively to pain or discomfort

Certain cultures discourage the expression of vulnerable feelings, especially in males. Be aware of this, and always treat each patient with dignity and respect.

There are things you can say or do to express your sensitivity to a patient who is feeling vulnerable. For example, leave the room when a patient is disrobing and knock on the door before reentering the room. If a patient feels uncomfortable discussing personal medical information with you, remind the patient that all information is confidential and won't be shared with anyone unless the third party is directly involved in the patient's medical care.

Managing Challenging Patients

Patients can present a challenge when they're angry, upset, or confused. Reasons for patient distress may include the following:

- prolonged waiting times
- financial issues
- illness, pain, or discomfort

Although it may be more difficult to deal with challenging patients, keep in mind that these patients deserve the same good customer service you provide to everyone else.

KEEP YOUR COOL

Even if you maintain a positive attitude, you may encounter a situation in which a patient becomes increasingly agitated. When a patient becomes confrontational, you must *always* remain professional. Focus your energy on remaining calm and controlled. Never yell at a patient or raise your voice. Arguing with a patient will only cause the patient to become defensive and increasingly frustrated.

Instead, learn how to keep your cool in tough situations.

1. First, take a minute to calm down and gather your thoughts.

2. Next, listen intently to what the patient is saying.

3. Then, address the patient in a polite but firm manner. Keep the volume of your voice at an appropriate level.

4. Finally, avoid telling the patient what he wants to hear just to quiet him down. Be sure the answer you provide is correct.

If you don't know the answer to a patient's question, find out the answer or refer the patient to a staff member who is qualified to answer the question.

Take a Time-out

Dealing with confrontational patients can drain your energy and your emotional reserves. You're probably familiar with your body's warning signs that let you know when you're starting to lose your composure. Your palms might become sweaty, and your heart might begin to beat faster. But before you react, decide to take a time-out and follow these suggestions.

- If possible, politely excuse yourself and put the phone down for a minute or step away from the front desk.

- Ask for assistance from a coworker.

- Breathe deeply and remind yourself that you're in control of the situation.

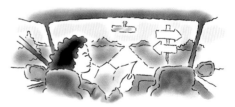

It helps to stop and gather your resources when you're not sure how to handle a difficult situation.

Be Polite but Firm

When you have to deliver disappointing news or refuse a patient's request, it's important to do so in a polite but firm manner. The following are examples of "dos" and "don'ts" to consider when dealing with patients who may be frustrated or upset.

Dos	Don'ts
Do be direct and assertive: "I'm sorry Mrs. Jones, but we can't accept this type of insurance."	*Don't* be aggressive: "Can't you read the posted sign? We don't accept this type of insurance."
Do offer your help: "I'm sorry you're in pain, Mr. Sanchez. Is there anything I can do to help you?"	*Don't* be uncaring or insensitive: "The pain should go away soon. Just sit here and wait for the physician."
Do give the patient choices: "I'm sorry for the inconvenience, but the physician is running behind schedule. You can reschedule your appointment or leave and return later if you'd like."	*Don't* take a power trip: "I'm not allowing you to see the physician. It's against office policy to place one patient ahead of another on the schedule."

DIFFICULT PATIENTS

Some patients seek attention by complaining or seem to always make "mountains out of molehills." Other patients might become angry about one thing when they're actually upset about something else. These patients can be difficult to handle. The following are examples of positive ways to deal with difficult patients.

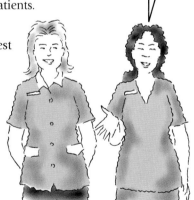

Sometimes, two people working together can solve the problem more efficiently and effectively.

- Be polite but firm.
- Let the patient know you care, but be honest about what you can do to help him.
- Keep a professional distance. Avoid becoming too emotionally involved in a patient's problems.
- Remember that the patient may get personal, but you should remain professional.
- Ask for help or advice from a coworker. You don't have to deal with difficult patients by yourself!

ANGRY OR HOSTILE PATIENTS

Here are some tips that will help you provide good customer service to patients who may be angry or hostile.

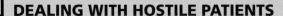

Ask The Professional | DEALING WITH HOSTILE PATIENTS

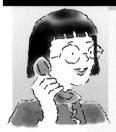

Q: *How do I know when a patient has crossed a line and has become threatening or aggressive?*

A: Trust your instincts! If the situation is getting out of hand, don't try to deal with it by yourself. Ask a coworker to help you calm the patient. Take all threats seriously. If the patient refuses to calm down or becomes aggressive or violent, then you may need to contact security or law enforcement. Don't escalate the problem by arguing with the patient. Ensure your safety and the safety of coworkers and patients.

- Listen! Listen! Listen! Move the patient into a quiet area instead of leaving him in the waiting room.
- Be supportive. Let the patient know you're here to help.
- Be open and honest in all communication.
- Never patronize the patient or belittle his concerns.
- Avoid giving false assurances.
- Ensure your own safety if the patient becomes threatening or aggressive.

CONFUSED PATIENTS

A patient may become confused if he has a cognitive impairment, such as dementia or Alzheimer disease. It's important to be sensitive to the needs of these patients; they may require additional assistance from you. (Helping patients with special needs is covered in greater detail in Chapter 4.)

Certain medications and other factors, such as illness, can also cause patients to become confused. Keep the following tips in mind when dealing with confused patients.

- Know your audience. Understand why the patient is confused and how this will affect your ability to provide high-quality customer service to the patient.
- Be a teacher. When giving information or instructions, always speak clearly and be specific.
- Have patience. A patient might need additional explanation or more time to process information. He may also be slower to respond.
- If the patient has a family member or caregiver present, include her in your interactions with the patient as well.

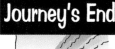

- Customer service is the quality of care you provide as a professional.
- In a health care setting, the patient is the customer. You determine patients' needs by communicating effectively and understanding how best to assist each patient.
- Providing good customer service is important because it helps you meet the health care needs of every patient.
- Make a good first impression on patients by developing a professional manner and image.

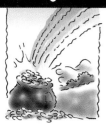

- A positive attitude can cultivate patient trust and prevent conflicts.
- Develop proper waiting room management techniques to maintain a positive and efficient work environment.
- Manage challenging patients by addressing their concerns, keeping them informed, and expressing your desire to help.
- Practice good customer service skills to keep the medical office running smoothly.

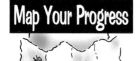

Answer the following multiple-choice questions.

1. Good *customer service* includes:
   a. being able to identify and help meet customers' needs.
   b. approaching difficult situations with a positive attitude.
   c. being competent and resourceful.
   d. all of the above

2. An example of a physiologic need is:
   a. safety.
   b. food.
   c. physical affection.
   d. trusting others.

3. As a medical assistant, how can you help patients meet their safety and security needs?
   a. by maintaining a sanitary work environment and practicing good personal hygiene
   b. by discussing with patients how their health concerns are affecting their overall wellness
   c. by treating patients with dignity and assisting them with a caring and empathetic attitude
   d. by helping patients meet small, realistic goals, such as following a physical therapy regimen

4. If a patient becomes confrontational, what might help you keep your composure?

    a. asking the patient to apologize
    b. giving in to the patient's requests
    c. taking a time-out to gather your thoughts
    d. ignoring the patient

5. *Diplomacy* is:
    a. handling people with graciousness and tact.
    b. reacting negatively to pain or discomfort.
    c. thinking about how you'd like to be treated as a patient.
    d. helping new patients become familiar with the office's policies.

6. When dealing with a confused patient, it's important to:
    a. understand why the patient is confused and how this will affect your ability to provide good customer service.
    b. use endearing terms, such as "honey" or "sweetie" to help the patient feel more at ease.
    c. move to a quiet area and speak to the patient's caregiver or family member in private.
    d. none of the above

7. What does it mean to respond empathetically to a patient?
    a. It means that you try to understand how a patient is feeling and why she's feeling that way.
    b. It means that you avoid confrontation with a patient at all costs.
    c. It means that you help a patient achieve self-actualization.
    d. It means that you don't get personally involved with a patient.

8. What is one way you can deal with angry patients properly?
    a. Be defensive when responding.
    b. Be open and honest when communicating.
    c. Be loud and attract a lot of attention.
    d. Be personable by talking about your own problems.

9. Why is it important to let a patient know if the physician is running behind schedule?
    a. so the patient can choose whether to reschedule his appointment or leave and return later
    b. so the patient doesn't become frustrated with the extended waiting time
    c. so the medical office runs smoothly
    d. all of the above

10. The responsibility of managing the waiting room includes:
    a. controlling the noise level in the front office.
    b. taking patients' vital signs.
    c. explaining basic medical procedures to patients.
    d. documenting the physician's instructions in patients' charts.

Chapter 4

DIVERSE UNIVERSE: EXPLORING CULTURAL DIVERSITY AND SPECIAL NEEDS

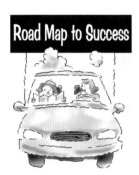

Road Map to Success

- Identify different cultures and some of their customs

- Explain how different customs can apply to health care

- Describe ways in which medical assistants can provide culturally sensitive care to patients

- Explain how to assist patients with special needs properly

- Explain how to care for geriatric patients properly

- Describe how to foster a trusting relationship with children and their parents

- Tailor your approach to patient education for patients from different cultures and those with specific needs

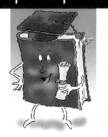

Chapter Competencies

- Be attentive, listen, and learn (ABHES 2.a.)

- Be courteous and diplomatic (ABHES 1.h.)

- Adapt what is said to the recipient's level of comprehension (ABHES 2.c.)

- Instruct individuals according to their needs (CAAHEP 3.c.3.b.)

- Be impartial and show empathy when dealing with patients (ABHES 2.b.)

- Adaptation for individualized needs (ABHES 2.m.)

In this chapter, you'll learn the importance of tailoring health care services to patients from different cultural backgrounds and with varying special needs. You'll also discover how patients' health care needs and expectations are influenced by their cultural backgrounds and unique conditions. You'll learn how to accommodate these needs with personalized and compassionate care. You'll explore the following topics as you read this chapter:

- cultural diversity—what it is and its impact on health care
- providing culturally conscious care
- the importance of learning about a patient's cultural background
- special needs—what they are and how they influence the health care you provide
- providing appropriate care to children and to older adults

Cultural Diversity

Culture is the shared beliefs, customs, and attitudes that provide social structure for daily living. Culture influences the roles and interactions within and between individuals, families, and communities. Individuals living in the same culture share many similarities with one another. For example, holding a door open for someone is considered a polite gesture. This is one of the unspoken "rules" of our culture that we all share. But do you know some of the ways in which we differ?

Cultural diversity refers to the differences that individuals and groups bring to a culture. In the medical office, you will encounter cultural diversity among patients as well as within the health care team. Being sensitive to the cultural customs, practices, and beliefs of others helps develop trust and understanding, which creates a more comfortable and productive work environment. You can learn to be sensitive to people's cultural differences by discovering how these differences influence and motivate people's actions and decisions.

The blending of different cultural backgrounds influences and changes the culture that we all share. So, why is cultural diversity an important thing to have?

APPRECIATING OUR DIFFERENCES

Imagine that every street in America looked exactly the same. How would our lives be different? We wouldn't travel anymore because we wouldn't be able tell one street from another! Just getting from one place to another would be a challenging task. Without differences, our world would start to feel small and boring because there would be little left to discover.

Thankfully, this isn't the case. We notice differences as we travel from state to state, town to town, and even while walking from block to block. Differences can make our lives feel fresh and exciting. We also notice differences among people, which make them more interesting. Cultural diversity refers to the ways in which people differ from one another, including:

Every snowflake is unique, just like each individual! Learn to appreciate our differences.

- racial classification
- national origin
- religious affiliation
- language
- physical size
- gender
- sexual orientation
- age
- disability
- socioeconomic status
- occupational status
- geographic location

HOW DOES CULTURAL DIVERSITY APPLY TO HEALTH CARE?

As a medical assistant, you'll care for many people from culturally diverse backgrounds. It's important that you understand how cultural beliefs, attitudes, and practices affect the health care needs of each patient. You should consider how the following cultural elements will affect patients' health care:

- genetic disposition to certain diseases or disorders
- cultural attitudes concerning pain and emotional expression
- cultural attitudes toward mental health
- gender roles and family support
- language barriers
- personal space needs
- socioeconomic level
- cultural attitudes concerning modesty
- differing views on illness and health care

Background and Genetics

A patient may be genetically predisposed to developing certain diseases or conditions because of her cultural background. For example, people of African, Hispanic, and Native American descent are more likely to develop diabetes than people of other ethnic backgrounds.

Once you begin working in a medical office, you'll become familiar with the different cultural backgrounds of patients seen in the office. With the physician's help, you can learn how to provide more targeted patient education. Patients may need to be informed of any genetic or cultural risk factors they possess and educated about how to decrease their risk level.

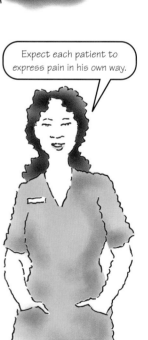

Being aware of the link between cultural background and certain diseases or conditions isn't just important for patients—it's important for you, too! By knowing about your own genetic risk factors, you can better monitor your health and wellness.

Reactions to Pain

Pain is a universal symptom, but the way a person expresses pain is often influenced by his cultural background. Some cultures allow for the open expression of emotional reactions to pain, whereas other cultures discourage expressing these feelings publicly. Be aware that the older generation can sometimes remain stoic when in pain due to previous hardships (for example, war, the Great Depression, etc.). You should be aware of culture's influence on patients when they're experiencing pain during procedures and examinations. Avoid assuming that because a patient isn't complaining about pain he isn't experiencing any. Medical assistants should be sensitive to the following signals of discomfort:

Expect each patient to express pain in his own way.

- holding, rubbing, or applying pressure to an area of the body
- self-restriction of activities that increase the pain
- uncontrollable and spontaneous expressions of discomfort, such as facial grimacing and moaning

Mental Health

Every cultural group has its own acceptable patterns of behavior regarding psychological well-being. What is considered "normal" can vary from group to group. Keep in mind that some patients may be reluctant to discuss their mental and emotional states with you, even though they may feel comfortable with you and trust your intentions.

Many ethnic groups are family-centered and wish to discuss their mental health only with the individuals closest to them. For example, members of Hispanic cultures often keep mental health problems within the family and would consider it inappropriate to discuss these problems with a stranger. According to traditional Chinese culture, mental illness is shameful, and seeking psychiatric help brings disgrace upon the family. Take into consideration a patient's cultural beliefs concerning mental illness before deciding to speak with her about her emotional well-being.

Gender Roles and Family Support

Cultural diversity includes smaller subgroups of people, such as families. Family dynamics often reflect cultural attitudes concerning gender roles and family support.

For example, in Islamic cultures, men are the heads of the household and make decisions for all family members. Women typically take a more passive role in these families. In other families, women are the dominant members. Or, men and women may share and exchange family roles frequently.

In other cultures, an individual's position within the family often determines her role. In these cultures, the elders (parents or grandparents) may make most of the important decisions for the other family members. The elders will often continue to make these decisions even after their children have become adults and have families of their own.

As a health care professional, you must be sensitive to the roles of each family member. For example, if a female patient's husband is asking all the questions or seems to be the only family member speaking, then it's safe to assume that he is the "spokesperson" for the family. As long as the patient doesn't object, you should be sure to include him in your conversations with the patient.

Language Barriers

Communication "roadblocks," such as language barriers between cultures, can also affect the health care patients receive. Language barriers include differences in:

- native or preferred language
- dialect
- pronunciation
- accent

Communication Strategies

You may encounter language barriers when interacting with patients from different cultural backgrounds and ethnicities. It's important to remember that even though you can't understand a patient, he still deserves your best care and attention. Here are some tips to help you communicate with non–English-speaking patients.

- Learn some basic phrases of the most common languages used in your area. (In several parts of the United States, this is some form of Spanish.) Patients will appreciate it if you try to communicate with them in their own language first. It shows initiative and interest.

- Be courteous and remember the importance of body language. Gestures and facial expressions can help you let the patient know that you're friendly and willing to help.

- Speak slowly and use simple words and phrases. A patient may understand some English. Read his body language for signals of understanding.

- Remember that an interpreter can help you communicate more effectively. Try to have the interpreter at the appointment if possible. (Translating services will be discussed later in this chapter.)

- Use flash cards and visual aids to get your message across. Pictures can help you explain a procedure or treatment when you're unable to communicate with words.

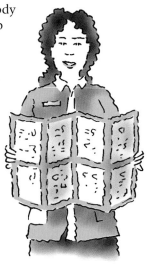

Visual Language Translator cards can help you explain something to a patient by using pictures instead of words.

The Benefits of Being Bilingual

As a medical assistant, you'll interact with patients from a variety of backgrounds every day. This is a situation in which being **bilingual,** or having the ability to speak and understand two languages, comes in handy. Speaking with a patient in her native language shows her that you value her culture and want to communicate more effectively with her. Being bilingual also helps you:

- provide care to patients from a variety of cultural backgrounds
- possibly draw new patients to the practice
- communicate more effectively, with fewer misunderstandings
- create a welcoming atmosphere
- act as a translator between patients and coworkers or physicians

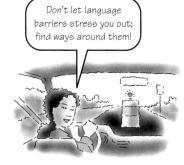

Don't let language barriers stress you out; find ways around them!

Personal Space

Our cultural experiences teach us that every individual has his own communication style. We learn to recognize and accept these differences as being a natural part of the person with whom we're speaking. For example, some people prefer to sit or stand close while interacting with others, and other people prefer to keep some distance between themselves and others. The amount of distance we prefer is often influenced by our culture's attitude regarding personal space.

As you learned in Chapter 2, personal space is the area around a person that is regarded as an extension of that person. We try not to enter another person's personal space unless we've been given some signal that permits us to do so. For example, you enter a patient's personal space when examining him or when providing therapeutic touch.

As a health care professional, you should be aware of the amount of personal space a patient requires. Respecting a patient's boundaries helps the patient feel secure and comfortable during her appointment. Some patients may be reassured by close inter-action, whereas others may feel threatened or upset. For example, people from many Hispanic cultures embrace physical closeness and may greet others warmly with a kiss on the cheek. A patient with this background may desire more therapeutic touch from you during particularly stressful moments during a procedure or examination. A more formal interaction, with less touch, might actually cause this patient stress or uneasiness. Remember to watch a patient's body language to gauge how she is feeling.

Socioeconomic Factors

A patient's economic status often affects how he meets his basic needs and maintains his health. Low income can affect the quality of a patient's health in several ways. Keep the following in mind when providing care.

- The patient may not be able to afford health insurance or may need financial assistance to pay medical fees.
- The patient may have a poor diet due to a low grocery bud-get. (Healthier food choices are often more expensive.)
- The patient may have a physically strenuous job that causes frequent health problems or disabilities.
- The patient may experience homelessness, causing stress and decreased ability to manage nutrition, hygiene, etc.

When helping a patient who is dealing with one or more of these problems, avoid making judgments. Instead, show empa-thy for the patient's situation and remember the importance

of impartiality. Professionalism requires that you treat each
patient with the same level of care and attention, regardless of his financial situation. You
can show initiative and professionalism by
researching local community resources to help
a patient meet his basic needs. Be familiar with
the locations of local shelters, free health care
clinics, and organizations that provide free meals.

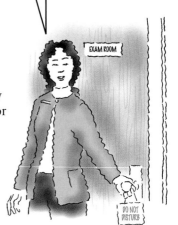

If a patient needs to undress before an
examination, respect his privacy by leaving
the room and closing the door.

Modesty Issues

The need for privacy and a sense of modesty can
vary from culture to culture. Many cultures follow
particular guidelines when it comes to exposing or
covering parts of the body. For example, a female
patient may refuse to be seen in a dressing gown
by a male nurse or physician. If you understand
that her culture doesn't allow physical contact
between strangers of the opposite sex, then you
will be sensitive to this issue and adjust your
care to meet the patient's cultural needs.

Other Issues

Every culture has its own view of illness and health care that can
vary according to spiritual and religious practices and beliefs.
Some cultures embrace the philosophies of Western medicine.
These patients will most likely seek standard Western treatment
options and physicians. However, other patients may hold values that are opposed to these philosophies and may seek out
alternative treatments and medicines.

Be aware of these differences and accommodate them as best
you can. For example, many Asian cultures believe that good
health is achieved through proper balance between yin and
yang. The proper balance between foods labeled as "hot" and
"cold" are believed to help maintain good health. Asking this
patient to make a change that may seem simple, such as modifying his diet in contradiction to these values, could have a poor
impact on his overall well-being. That's why health care providers need to consider patients' cultural values and practices when
prescribing or implementing treatment plans.

Providing Culturally Conscious Care

As a medical assistant, you'll need to be sensitive to each patient's
cultural background, values, and beliefs when you're providing
care. As you will see, you can learn to provide culturally conscious
care by doing the following:

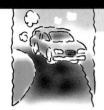

Road Rules

CULTURAL DIVERSITY AND THE MEDICAL ASSISTANT

It's important to be sensitive to cultural diversity in the medical office. Cultural diversity is multilayered and serves several functions in a person's life. In the health care setting:

- A patient's diet and nutrition is a vital component of her health care. A patient's genetics can also predispose her to certain medical diseases or disorders.

- Everyone feels pain, but culture influences how people choose to express pain. Watch for discrepancies between how a patient says she feels and what her body language is telling you.

- Gender roles and family dynamics can shape how a person receives and experiences health care.

- Becoming bilingual can be an advantage when interacting with non–English-speaking patients.

- The amount of personal space a patient requires often depends on the patient's cultural attitudes concerning space and touch, as well as personal preferences.

- The amount of money a person has can affect her ability to maintain good health. Be sensitive to the socioeconomic factors that can contribute to poor health in patients.

- Although one patient may be completely at ease with having to undress for a physical examination, another patient may be extremely uncomfortable. Be aware of the various cultural attitudes and personal preferences regarding modesty.

- Patients' spiritual and religious practices can influence their attitudes toward health care. When possible, accommodate these differences.

- becoming culturally self-aware
- avoiding ethnocentrism, stereotypes, and bias
- having a desire to learn about patients' cultures
- finding ways to accommodate patients' values and practices when providing care

BE SELF-AWARE

Part of providing culturally conscious care is the ability to understand how cultural influences affect your own life. Take an objective look at your own beliefs, values, practices, and family experiences. How do these factors influence your own health care needs? As you become more sensitive to the importance of culturally conscious health care in your own life, you'll be able to acknowledge cultural influences in patients' lives. You'll also find ways in which you can accommodate a patient's cultural background when providing care.

AVOID ETHNOCENTRISM

All cultural traditions, beliefs, and practices hold value. However, placing too much emphasis on the importance of your own cultural background can

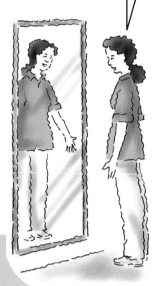

By taking a good look at your own cultural beliefs, values, and practices, you'll become more sensitive to the cultural influences in patients' lives.

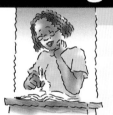

Travelog DEVELOPING CULTURAL SELF-AWARENESS

I didn't understand how a patient's cultural background could affect his health care until I looked at my own values and practices. In my Southern, African American family, we attend church every Sunday and then cook a big meal and eat together as a family. The foods we choose and the ways in which we prepare them aren't always healthy, but these family meals are important to us because they're part of a long tradition.

When I visited my physician recently, he told me that my blood pressure was high and asked me to modify my diet. I couldn't imagine giving up all the foods I loved! I explained to him the significance that soul food had in my life. He explained that most of the foods I enjoy can be part of a healthy diet if I consume them in moderation. He worked with me to develop a diet and exercise plan that fits my lifestyle.

This experience helped me realize how important our cultural values and practices really are. Now when I interact with patients, I'm more sensitive to the ways in which their own culture affects their health care needs!

lead to **ethnocentrism,** or the belief that one's own ideas, beliefs, and practices are superior and preferable to others. You can avoid ethnocentrism by becoming self-aware and understanding health and illness from the perspective of the patient receiving care. Pushing your beliefs and values on a patient is never acceptable. If a patient feels that you respect his beliefs, you'll be more likely to earn his trust.

AVOID STEREOTYPING AND BIAS

As a medical assistant, you'll interact with patients from various walks of life. Some patients may hold personal values that are very different from your own. However, you must avoid letting your personal values or **biases** (opinions) influence the quality of health care you provide to a patient. All patients must be treated fairly, respectfully, and with dignity, regardless of their personal values. To treat patients in any other way is **discrimination.**

Stereotyping is holding an opinion of all members of a particular culture or group based on oversimplified or negative characterizations. We sometimes stereotype other people when we misunderstand them or feel threatened or frightened by their differences. Stereotypes lead us to judge people before we've gotten to know them.

Because stereotypes are based on false assumptions about a group, never use them to influence how a patient should be treated. By being impartial, you show patients that you accept all human differences as a part of life and want to provide equal health care for everyone.

HAVE A DESIRE TO LEARN

Television, the Internet, and other media bombard our screens with cultural misrepresentations and stereotypes every day. So how do you "unlearn" a personal bias or stereotype? Well, one important way is by talking to people! Patients will respond positively if they sense that you're sincerely interested in their cultural background and beliefs. Here are some tips to remember when learning about patients:

- Get to know your patients and the cultural groups that are specific to your community. Attend events that encourage cultural diversity education and discussion.

- Practice your listening and observation skills to acquire knowledge of the beliefs and practices of the patients you care for.

- When asking a patient about his culture, approach the topic with sensitivity. Build trust between you and the patient before asking about his cultural associations.
- Remember that it's better to ask a patient about his culture than to make assumptions or judgments.

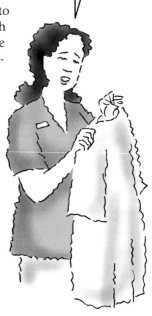

"One size fits all"? When it comes to providing health care, a tailored approach is best!

Many groups, especially minorities, have been made to feel devalued and stereotyped by society. If you approach a patient with an open mind and empathetic attitude, he will likely feel more comfortable sharing his cultural values with you.

BE ACCOMMODATING

Ask the patient if he has any special requests regarding his health care. A patient may tell you up front if he has any deeply held values, beliefs, or practices that might conflict with the care you'd normally provide. Try to accommodate these needs by modifying your behavior, and inform the physician if you feel that the treatment plan may need to be modified as well.

For example, if a patient is fasting for religious purposes, allow for this special circumstance. Don't pressure the patient into eating or drinking anything. Respecting the patient's right to cultural practices is an important part of providing culturally conscious care.

Cultural Practices

It's essential to take into account a patient's cultural background when providing health care. It's equally important to incorporate the patient's cultural practices whenever possible, as long as those practices aren't harmful or dangerous to the patient's health. For example, if a patient traditionally drinks an herbal tea to alleviate symptoms of an illness, both the herbal tea and prescribed medications may be used. As long as the tea is safe to drink and the ingredients don't interfere with the action of the medication, it's perfectly acceptable to incorporate this cultural practice. To ignore or disregard a patient's cultural practices may upset the patient and result in his refusal to receive care or follow treatment plans. You can serve patients by embracing their cultural traditions and practices.

However, there are situations where health care professionals are unable to accommodate a patient's cultural practices. For example, if a patient has been fasting for an extended period of time and his health is in danger, the physician might advise against continuing the fast. Likewise, if a patient's cultural background dictates that he can't take any medications, the physician might advise against such a practice.

In most cases, patients have the final say about what care they will accept and which treatment plans they will follow. The only exceptions to this rule are patients who are minors (unless they are emancipated minors) and patients who lack the mental competence to make their own health care decisions. When a patient chooses to act against the physician's medical advice, the patient's refusal should be recorded in his medical record. Documentation of patient refusal is important because, if the patient's condition worsens or he dies, there may be legal consequences for the physician.

Family Roles

Keep in mind that, in some families, one person makes most of the health care decisions for all family members. Often, the patient will seek this family member's approval before accepting a treatment plan. With the patient's permission, you can involve the dominant family member in the patient's health care to avoid conflict. The patient will also be more likely to follow the treatment plan if the dominant family member agrees with it.

DON'T FORCE IT

Keep in mind that health care practices are a part of cultural attitudes and beliefs. Because of this connection, health care practices are adjusted as the culture changes.

For example, if a patient is following a potentially harmful health practice for cultural reasons, the physician will decide if

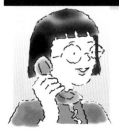

Ask The Professional **ACCOMMODATING PATIENTS**

Q: *How can I accommodate patients who aren't the decision makers in their family?*

A: Patients who don't make their own health care decisions may seem reluctant to offer suggestions or information. Ask to speak with the decision maker directly, in the presence of the patient. Make sure that you explain all information thoroughly and accurately to both individuals. The patient may want to discuss the information with the decision maker in private.

a change in the treatment plan is necessary. In this situation, remember that you need to support the patient. Never try to force the patient to participate in care that opposes her personal values. If the patient is forced to accept care or treatment, she may experience feelings of guilt or shame that can put her well-being at greater risk. Instead, work with the physician to develop a treatment plan that works cooperatively with the patient's values and belief systems.

> Don't force it! When possible, work with the physician to accommodate a patient's cultural beliefs and personal values.

GET HELP

If the physician is having difficulty developing acceptable treatment or care options, work with her to seek outside help from a patient's family members, clergy, or traditional healers. Acknowledging the patient's need for health care that corresponds with his cultural values is a good way to build trust. The patient will be more likely to accept your services if you've established a desire to be cooperative and empathetic.

CULTURAL AWARENESS SELF-ASSESSMENT

How culturally aware are you? Are there areas where you need improvement? Take this short self-assessment to find out!

Directions: Enter Y for "yes" or N for "no" for each item:

____ I believe that all patients should be treated with respect for their culture, even though it may be different from my own.

____ I don't impose my beliefs and values onto patients or their family members.

____ I believe it's OK to speak a language other than English.

____ I'm aware that the roles family members play may differ according to culture.

____ I understand that male-female roles may vary among different cultures and ethnic groups, and I recognize and respect the designated decision maker in each family.

____ For patients and families who speak languages other than my own, I'll try to learn and use key words in their language so I can communicate with them better.

___ I understand that people who have limited English skills have the same intellectual capacity as anyone else and may be very capable of communicating clearly in their own language.

___ I recognize that the meaning or value of medical treatment and health education may vary greatly among cultures.

___ I understand that religion and other beliefs may affect how patients and families respond to illness, disease, and death.

___ I recognize that culture may influence verbal and non-verbal communication in many ways, including eye contact, personal space, asking and responding to questions, and comfort with silence.

___ I believe that posters, magazines, and brochures in the medical office should be of interest to and reflect the different cultures of patients and families served by a medical practice.

___ I think it's important to stay up-to-date on major health concerns and issues for the different ethnic groups living in the area served by a medical office.

If you answered "yes" for most questions, congratulations! Your cultural awareness is in great shape! If not, you might need to examine some of your opinions so they don't affect your ability to provide quality, culturally conscious care to all patients.

Adapted from Goode TD. Promoting cultural competence and cultural diversity in early intervention and early childhood settings (Washington, DC: Georgetown University Center for Child and Human Development, 1989, revised 2002).

Caring for Patients with Special Needs

Caring for patients with special needs requires patience and sensitivity. **Special needs** are medical conditions that require special care and consideration from medical staff, family members, and others. Acquiring the appropriate knowledge and skills is essential to meeting the needs of patients with special needs, such as:

- developmental (physical and mental) disabilities
- mental illnesses

- dementia
- hearing impairments
- sight impairments
- mobility challenges
- communicable infections
- cancer

PATIENTS WITH DEVELOPMENTAL DISABILITIES

Developmental disabilities are permanent disabilities that affect people before they reach adulthood. These disabilities interfere with a person's ability to reach developmental milestones, such as walking or talking. A developmental disability can affect a person's mental functioning, physical functioning, or both. Some disabilities are mild (e.g., the person is able to live independently after reaching adulthood), whereas others are more severe (e.g., the person requires total care).

Some common developmental disabilities include autism, cerebral palsy, and Down syndrome.

Autism

A 2007 report conducted by the Centers for Disease Control and Prevention found that 1 in 150 children in America have some form of **autism**. This disability affects normal functioning of the brain. Although the specific cause of autism is unknown, researchers suspect a genetic link. The signs of autism usually appear by the time a child is three years old.

Autism is a *spectrum* disorder, meaning it affects each person differently and at various levels of severity. People with autism sometimes suffer from other disorders as well, such as mental retardation and seizure disorders. However, many people with autism have average or above-average intelligence.

People with autism often have difficulty communicating with and relating to other people and their surroundings. They tend to respond to information in unique ways. Some individuals have delays in language and difficulty starting and maintaining a conversation. Other traits people with autism can display include:

- insisting on repetition and resisting change
- repeating words or phrases instead of using normal, responsive language
- laughing (and/or crying) for no apparent reason; showing distress for reasons not apparent to others

- having a preference for being alone; acting distant or detached
- making little or no eye contact
- being unresponsive to normal teaching methods
- having an obsessive attachment to objects
- seeming overly sensitive (or hardly sensitive at all) to pain
- not possessing any real fear of danger
- being physically overactive or underactive
- not responding to verbal cues; acting as if deaf even though the patient's hearing is intact

> When caring for a patient with autism, take cues from the parent or caregiver to determine the best way to approach the patient.

Cerebral Palsy

Cerebral palsy affects a person's motor control; it is sometimes accompanied by mental retardation. Cerebral palsy can be **congenital** (meaning a person is born with it) or caused by a brain injury that occurs either during birth or in early childhood. The degree of disability varies from person to person. Cerebral palsy can affect body movements in two different ways.

- One type of cerebral palsy causes spasms and shortening of the muscles, which can affect a person's ability to walk and perform basic self-care tasks.
- Another type of cerebral palsy can cause a person's arms, legs, and parts of the upper body (including facial muscles) to move involuntarily.

Down Syndrome

People born with this genetic disorder have an extra chromosome, which causes mental retardation and muscle weakness. Approximately 1 in every 1,000 children is born with **Down syndrome.** People with Down syndrome often share certain physical characteristics, such as almond-shaped eyes and short stature. Many people with Down syndrome are also born with heart defects, which can be corrected with surgery or medication. Because Down syndrome can affect the muscles used for breathing, frequent respiratory tract infections are also common.

Down syndrome is accompanied by some degree of mental retardation, although many adults with Down syndrome live independently and have jobs. Group homes give people with Down syndrome the opportunity to live on their own in a supervised and supportive environment.

Providing Care

As a medical assistant, it's likely that you'll encounter patients who have developmental disabilities. Remember, these patients have the same physical and emotional needs as everyone else. For example, they need to maintain a healthy diet and exercise regularly. They also need to feel loved and cared for. However, patients with developmental disabilities often have other special needs that need to be met as well.

When working with a patient who has a developmental disability, the care you provide must be specific to the person's abilities and disabilities. Because each person is affected differently, learn as much as you can about each patient you see in the medical office. Focus on the patient's abilities so you can provide compassionate and appropriate care.

Communicating: Get Creative!

Developmental disabilities often affect communication skills. Some people are unable to speak or learn language skills due to a lack of motor skills, mental capabilities, or both. Certain disorders, such as cerebral palsy, are sometimes accompanied by vision or hearing problems, which also hinder communication.

Because of these difficulties, people with developmental disabilities often rely on other ways of communicating. For example, they may find it easier to communicate in nonverbal ways, such as through facial expressions, gestures, and body language. Follow the tips below to improve your communication with these patients.

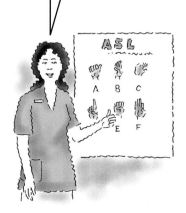

Some patients with developmental disabilities communicate with sign language. Learn a few basic signs so you can communicate with patients in their own language.

- Ask patients' caregivers or family members which communication methods work best.

- When speaking with patients who have mental disabilities, use simple words and short phrases. Be sure to give patients enough time to process what you're saying.

- When possible, ask questions that can be answered with a simple "yes" or "no" to make it easier for patients to respond.

- Communicate your care and compassion for patients by using therapeutic touch (when appropriate) and kind, encouraging words.

PATIENTS WITH MENTAL ILLNESSES

Mental illnesses, also called mental disorders, are psychological disorders that affect a person's thought processes, emotions, or behavior. Common mental illnesses include depression, anxiety, and bipolar disorder. Most mental illnesses can be controlled and treated with medications and other therapies. In fact, in recent times, researchers have discovered a lot of new information about mental illnesses. Advances in neuroscience (the study of the brain and nervous system) and psychology have shed light on mental illnesses, their causes, and treatment options.

However, a cultural bias still exists against people with mental illnesses. They are often incorrectly labeled as lazy or attention seeking. These biases can cause people suffering from mental illness to feel ashamed and guilty—even to resist seeking treatment. The truth is that mental illness is a day-to-day reality for many people in our culture. Occurrences of mental illness are on the rise and should be addressed as a serious health concern.

Mental illness can be long-term or short-term. It can have roots in an individual's genetics or background, or it may be circumstantial. For example, a patient can experience a traumatic event that pushes her toward mental illness, especially if she is genetically predisposed to depression and anxiety. A patient will need your support when a mental illness appears or worsens. Here are a few suggestions for helping patients who have mental illnesses.

- Keep the patient informed. Tell her, "I'm going to touch your arm now," or "This will just take a minute." Informing the patient will help her feel secure and comfortable.
- Keep conversations focused and professional.
- Never force or demand answers from patients who are withdrawn or mute.
- Avoid confirming hearing voices or seeing nonexistent objects.
- If you ever feel unsafe with a patient, tell your supervisor or get help.
- Remember to be professional and nonjudgmental at all times.

PATIENTS WITH DEMENTIA

Dementia is a progressive and permanent loss of the ability to think and remember, caused by damage to the brain tissue. Dementia affects a patient's mental and physical abilities, so everyday activities such as bathing, dressing, and eating can become very challenging. Patients with dementia often forget how to do things. As a result, they may become angry or frustrated with themselves or other people. Follow these suggestions when assisting patients with dementia.

- Ask the patient's family members how best to communicate with the patient, especially with someone who has advanced dementia.
- Speak clearly and in a calm tone of voice.
- Consider using gentle therapeutic touch. Many people with dementia respond positively to touch.
- Remind the person what to do at each step of the examination or procedure.
- Allow the patient to do as much for himself as possible; this boosts self-esteem.
- Use gestures along with spoken instructions. For example, if the patient needs to be seated on the examination table, you might say, "Mrs. Rodriguez, come sit here, please" and motion to the examination table with your hand.
- Plan for the treatment or procedure in advance. Being prepared and having everything you need may decrease the time it takes to complete each task, which will reduce the stress level of patients with dementia.

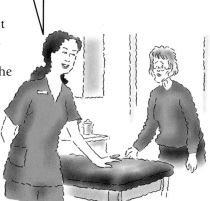

When caring for patients who suffer from dementia, remember to use gestures along with spoken instructions.

PATIENTS WITH HEARING IMPAIRMENTS

There are many types of hearing impairments. Impairments can range from partial hearing loss to **anacusis,** or complete hearing loss. Some patients were born hearing impaired, and others may have suffered hearing loss as a result of an accident, injury, or illness.

Most patients with anacusis are experts at communicating through sign language, interpreters, lip reading, or other methods. Patients with partial hearing loss, however, may have a more difficult time communicating. Patients suffering from partial hearing loss can often benefit from hearing aids and other devices. Consider the following suggestions when providing care for hearing-impaired patients:

- Talk directly to the patient, and make sure she can see your facial expressions and gestures.
- Talk to the patient in a quiet, distraction-free area.
- Make sure the room is well-lit. Often, hearing-impaired patients will rely more heavily upon their sense of sight.
- Lower the pitch of your voice, but don't whisper. Speak with force and pronounce each syllable distinctly. Shouting won't help the patient understand you.
- Use shorter phrases and sentences.
- Use diagrams or other visual aids to help a patient understand your message and intent.
- If the patient is accompanied by a family member or caregiver, work with the patient's family member to ensure understanding.

PATIENTS WITH SIGHT IMPAIRMENTS

Sight impairments can range from complete blindness to blurred vision. Like hearing impairments, sight impairments can occur naturally or may be a result of an accident or health problem. The following are some common medical conditions that can cause sight impairments:

- cataract
- hyperopia (farsightedness)
- glaucoma
- myopia (nearsightedness)
- nyctalopia (night blindness)
- presbyopia (inability to focus sharply)
- retinal detachment

Often, the patient will experience a gradual loss of vision. Nonverbal messages (such as gestures and facial expressions) are often lost when communicating with sight-impaired patients. So, it's necessary to find alternative ways of communicating with these patients. Effective communication will help you provide better care. Here are several tips to follow when interacting with sight-impaired patients.

- Identify yourself by name when you or the patient enters the room.
- Avoid raising your voice; being sight-impaired doesn't affect a patient's hearing.
- Talk to the patient about the procedure and what you're doing as you perform each step.

- Help the patient become familiar with her surroundings by having her touch a table, chair, or other object in the room.
- Assist the patient by offering an arm or hand.
- Tell the patient when you'll be leaving the room and knock before entering.
- Explain the reason for other sounds, such as procedural equipment and machines.

> Patients with sight loss often rely on their hearing, so speak clearly and directly to these patients.

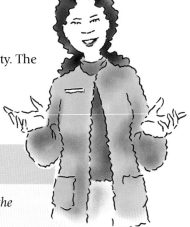

PATIENTS WITH MOBILITY CHALLENGES

Some diseases and conditions can impair mobility. The following are several examples.

- **Muscular dystrophy** is an inherited disease that causes the skeletal muscles to

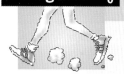

Running Smoothly

SERVICE ANIMALS

What if a patient brings a service animal into the medical office?

Suppose a patient brings his seeing-eye dog to his appointment. He asks if he can keep the dog with him in the office. What would you say?

The Americans with Disabilities Act (ADA) forbids businesses from banning service animals. A **service animal** is any animal that has been trained to provide assistance to a person with a disability. Some examples of the tasks performed by service animals include:

- alerting the disabled person to sounds
- picking up items
- pulling wheelchairs
- sensing smells

The service animal should not be separated from its owner and should enter the examination room with the patient. The ADA law takes precedence over local health department laws banning animals in health care facilities.

Remember that these animals are working, and some patients don't like it when people pet the work animals or give them treats. It's always a good idea to ask before petting a work animal.

weaken. There are several types of muscular dystrophy. Two common types, Duchenne muscular dystrophy and Becker muscular dystrophy, first affect a child's ability to walk and later affect the muscles in the arms and diaphragm as well.

- **Paralysis** can result from many different diseases that affect either the muscles or the brain. People with paralysis can have impaired movement or a complete loss of voluntary muscle movement in certain parts of the body.

- **Multiple sclerosis (MS)** is a disorder that affects the nervous system. MS progresses at different rates, depending on the individual. The nerves in the hands, feet, and eyes are usually affected before the central nervous system is affected. MS can cause muscle weakness and eventual paralysis.

When providing care to patients who have mobility challenges, it's necessary to consider each patient's individual abilities and disabilities. For example, some young patients with muscular dystrophy may be able to walk with the help of leg braces or a walker, whereas other patients may be confined to wheelchairs. Similarly, patients can experience mild to severe paralysis, depending on the disease or condition from which they suffer.

Remember to be patient and allow patients to complete the tasks they're able to complete. However, if you notice, for example, that a patient is having difficulty walking, offer your assistance. Likewise, you may need to assist a patient with positioning during physical examinations. By paying attention to each patient's specific needs, you'll be able to provide customized care.

PATIENTS WITH COMMUNICABLE INFECTIONS

As a medical assistant, you'll probably encounter patients with communicable infections on a daily basis. **Communicable infections** are infections that can be spread from one person to another. Some communicable infections, such as the common cold, can be transmitted through casual contact. For example, you can get a cold just by touching a doorknob after someone who has a cold has touched it or by sitting next to someone with a cold in a crowded waiting room. Other infections, such as hepatitis and AIDS, can only be transmitted through the exchange of blood or body fluids.

The Chain of Infection

For an infection to spread from one person to another, it must pass through the six links in the **chain of infection.**

1. First, a *pathogen* must be present. A pathogen is a microbe, or germ, that causes illness.

2. Next, the pathogen must be stored in a suitable *reservoir,* such as a human, an animal, food, water, milk, or an object or surface that has come in contact with an infected person's body fluids.

3. The reservoir needs to have a *portal of exit* so the pathogen can leave the reservoir. In humans, common portals of exit include the digestive tract (through saliva), the respiratory tract (through mucus), and the skin (through blood or other drainage from wounds).

4. Then, the pathogen must have a *method of transmission.* Direct transmission occurs when a noninfected person has contact with an infected person. For example, when a person with a cold sneezes, a noninfected person might inhale droplets from the infected person. Indirect transmission occurs when a noninfected person comes in contact with an object or surface that has been **contaminated** (soiled) by pathogens.

5. Next, a *portal of entry* must be available. In humans, pathogens can enter the body through portals such as the respiratory, digestive, and reproductive systems or though a break in the skin.

6. Finally, there must be a *susceptible host.* Harmful microbes enter the human body all the time, but the body's defense systems can fight off most of these pathogens. However, some people with weakened or undeveloped immune systems are at greater risk for infection. At-risk patients include young children, older adult patients, patients who have poor general health, and patients who suffer from high levels of stress and fatigue.

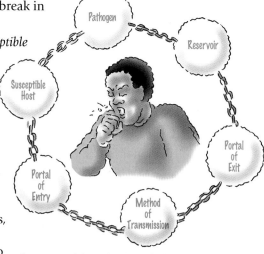

There are six links in the chain of infection. A pathogen must pass through each link for an infection to spread from one person to another.

Breaking the Chain

So, how can you control the spread of infection in the medical office? You can follow safety practices, called **infection control,** to ensure that patients with communicable infections don't pass them on to other patients or staff members. Follow these tips to help "break the chain" of infection.

- Wash your hands often. Remember to wash them when you first arrive at the office; after using the bathroom; before handling food or drink; and after coughing, sneezing, or blowing your nose. You should also wash your hands before and after any contact with a patient, even if you were wearing gloves.
- Keep contaminated or dirty items, such as used linens, away from your clothing.
- Follow office procedures for disposing of used gowns and linens or preparing them for the laundry.
- Dispose of trash, medical waste, and sharps in the proper receptacles.
- When necessary, wear **personal protective equipment (PPE),** such as disposable gloves, gowns, masks, and protective eyewear. PPE is usually required any time you might come in contact with a patient's body fluids or substances.
- Use precautions with patients who have communicable infections. For example, if a patient suspects that he has the flu, it may be necessary to have him wait for the physician in a private examination room instead of in the waiting room. Following these precautions will decrease the risk of the patient's transmitting the infection to other patients.

PATIENTS WITH CANCER

Patients with cancer also have special physical needs that must be met. Depending on the type of cancer a person has and the method(s) of treatment being used, the patient may be experiencing side effects. Some common side effects of radiation therapy (which involves the use of x-ray beams to destroy the cancer cells) and chemotherapy (which involves the use of medications) include:

- digestive problems, such as nausea, vomiting, loss of appetite, and diarrhea
- skin irritation and skin breakdown
- fatigue
- increased risk for infection

The physician may prescribe treatments for these side effects. For example, skin breakdown can be prevented with gentle, thorough skin care. Patients can fight fatigue and maintain muscle strength with mild exercise combined with periods of rest.

As a medical assistant, however, you can do your part to help with other side effects, such as patients' increased risk for infection. Because some cancer treatments affect the body's ability to fight off infections, these patients have an increased risk for contracting communicable infections. Even less serious infections, such as the common cold or the flu, can turn into pneumonia. For this reason, it's especially important to protect cancer patients from infection. Be careful to follow all infection control procedures, such as washing your hands often and wearing PPE. Whenever possible, allow these patients to wait for the physician in a private examination room. By minimizing the time they spend in the waiting room, you'll be helping to minimize their risk for infection.

Caring for Geriatric Patients

Assisting geriatric patients during examinations and procedures can present several unique challenges. As a medical assistant, you'll need to be aware of issues such as:

- decreased mobility
- the effects of aging on the body
- concurrent illnesses (two or more illnesses that occur at the same time)
- *polypharmacy* (the patient may be taking many different medications)

For example, an older adult patient may have decreased mobility. It may be a struggle just for the patient to arrive for his scheduled appointments on time. His body is slowing down, and he may walk slowly and with less ease. It's important to have patience when caring for geriatric patients. As a medical assistant, you may be asked to assist a patient when walking, standing, or sitting. Additionally, the patient may need help undressing or getting up on the exam table. Always offer help, as this gives patients the opportunity to accept assistance without having to ask for it.

Older adult patients may also be feeling the effects of aging on their bodies. They may have concurrent illnesses that slow down the recovery process, such as diabetes and cardiovascular disease. Concurrent illnesses also make differentiating signs and symptoms difficult. You might ask the patient specific questions, such as "When did this symptom develop?" Asking specific questions makes it easier for the physician to rule out possible causes and to detect other illnesses.

Because some older adult patients often experience several illnesses at the same time, they are more likely to be taking multiple medications. This can cause problems for a patient if he has trouble remembering when to take certain medications. Also, certain combinations of medications may be harmful if taken together. (Educating older adult patients about medication is discussed later in this chapter.)

You can help care for older adult patients by:

- reinforcing medical compliance
- reinforcing mental health
- helping patients cope with aging
- being familiar with the signs and symptoms of common diseases
- recognizing elder abuse and neglect

REINFORCING MEDICAL COMPLIANCE IN OLDER ADULTS

To help older adults patients comply with the physician's instructions, follow these tips.

- Write down instructions in laymen's terms.
- Use large, clear print.
- Ask the patient to repeat instructions so it's clear to you that she understands them.
- Give the patient a copy of a large appointment calendar and list the times and dates of appointments, scheduled procedures, and medications.

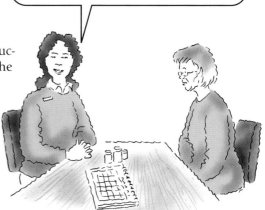

When educating older adult patients about their medications, remember to be patient! Ask the patient to repeat instructions back to you, and take the time to address any questions the patient may have.

REINFORCING MENTAL HEALTH IN OLDER ADULTS

How healthy a person feels depends on his overall wellness. Wellness not only involves the health of a person's physical body; it's also determined by mental and emotional health.

Chronic physical problems can eventually lead to a decline in mental and emotional wellness.

Reasons why older adult patients can suffer from mental and emotional problems include:

- struggling to adapt to a new role in life (retirement, fewer social interactions, etc.)
- a loss of independence due to the need to rely upon others for basic care
- an increased number of health problems that can decrease physical activity
- a loss of companionship and support

Older adult patients who face these challenges often experience painful feelings of loss, anger, and sadness. A patient may have no one to vent these feelings to or may receive hostile or apathetic responses from others. In cases such as this, you may be the "safe" person with whom the patient feels comfortable sharing his frustrations. For these reasons, it's essential to create an environment that fosters emotional openness and compassion. Follow these guidelines when reinforcing mental health in the older adults.

- Listen to and support the patient. Help him cope with and express his feelings. Let the patient talk openly about topics such as illness and death.
- Remember that all emotions are acceptable. Let the patient be honest about how he's feeling. If the patient isn't allowed to feel "negative" emotions, like sadness or anger, then he won't be able to work through them to see things in a more positive light.
- Maintain open communication. Offer advice and encouragement without diagnosing or providing false reassurances.
- Help the patient maintain positive self-esteem. Focus on the patient's positive qualities and abilities. It never hurts to give a sincere compliment!

HELPING PATIENTS COPE WITH AGING

The aging process can be stressful for individuals, especially if they are experiencing additional challenges, such as financial instability and health problems. Older adult patients often experience a sense of loss, and rightfully so. An older adult patient may be suffering the loss or change of:

- senses (such as sight and hearing)
- mobility and independence

- clarity of perception
- employment
- home
- spouse
- friends

It's also important to be aware of the more abstract losses. These losses can cause just as much grief as the visible losses and include:

- life purpose
- goals
- a sense of achievement
- self-worth
- motivation
- recognition
- security

Part of providing excellent care to older adult patients is finding ways to help them cope with the aging process. These losses can foster feelings of helplessness and personal insignificance within the individual. To lessen these feelings, involve older adult patients in their own health care as much as possible by allowing them to have a voice in decisions that will affect their care. You can also help older adult patients by taking the following actions.

> Talk to older adult patients about their feelings concerning aging. Do they need some extra help coping?

- Listen closely to their fears and concerns. A patient may just need someone to talk to.
- Respect each patient's right to these feelings. Avoid judging a patient's feelings or minimizing their importance.
- Help patients reduce the stressors in their lives. Offering solutions such as adopting a pet may help decrease tension and promote good health and wellness.
- Identify community resources, such as local Meals on Wheels programs, and help older adult patients obtain these services.
- Take note of changes in health and wellness that should be mentioned to the physician or documented in patients' medical records.

COMMON DISEASES OF OLDER ADULTS

When caring for older adult patients, keep in mind that there are several diseases specific to these patients.

If you're aware of the risk for these diseases, you'll be alert to the signs and symptoms. Be sure to notify the physician if a patient's health or behavior changes. Some of the common diseases among older adult patients include:

- Parkinson disease
- Alzheimer disease
- heart disease
- chronic obstructive pulmonary disease (COPD)
- pneumonia
- stroke
- diabetes

Parkinson Disease

Parkinson disease is a slow, progressive neurological disease that affects the brain cells that produce the neurotransmitter dopamine. With lower levels of dopamine, a patient experiences involuntary muscle movements and the inability to control these movements. The disease may progress over ten years or longer before resulting in complete debilitation or death. These are the signs and symptoms of Parkinson disease:

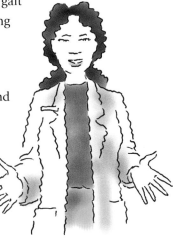

Know the signs of Parkinson disease so that you can alert the physician to potential concerns for the patient.

- muscle rigidity
- abnormally slow voluntary movements
- difficulty walking, or walking with a shuffling gait
- forward-bending posture and lack of arm swing
- laryngeal rigidity and monotone voice
- pharyngeal rigidity with **dysphagia** (difficulty swallowing) and drooling
- facial muscle rigidity, with expressionless face and infrequent blinking reflex
- small tremors in fingers

Parkinson disease currently has no cure. The diagnosis of Parkinson disease is usually made by excluding other causes. Treatment includes medication and a procedure known as *deep brain stimulation* to reduce tremors and rigidity.

Alzheimer Disease

Dementia in older adults is often attributed to Alzheimer disease. The symptoms of Alzheimer disease may appear in

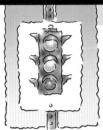

Signs & Signals

HELPING PATIENTS COPE WITH PARKINSON DISEASE

Patients who suffer from Parkinson disease retain their cognitive abilities and are aware of (and often embarrassed by) the outward signs of their disease. As a result, patients can become easily depressed and isolated. They require additional care and support from you, their family and friends, and outside support groups. As a medical assistant, there are several things you can do to help patients suffering from Parkinson disease:

- Promote their independence.
- Listen to patients. Their cognitive abilities are intact and require stimulation.
- Educate patients about safety risks. The forward-bending posture and altered gait can cause frequent falls. Encourage the patient to hold onto railings and to remove rugs and loose cords from the home to prevent accidental tripping.
- Enlist the help of local support groups.
- Improve the patient's quality of life through education. For example, the physician may ask you to explain to a patient how to reduce his symptoms by increasing fluid intake, eating a balanced diet, and increasing fiber intake.

patients as young as 40 years old and may worsen as the disease progresses. Symptoms of Alzheimer disease include:

- memory loss
- forgetfulness
- disorientation
- dementia
- loss of ability to care for oneself
- loss of speech
- loss of control of basic body functions
- feelings of anger, hostility, confusion, and frustration

Alzheimer disease has several recognized stages. The progression from one stage to the next may be very gradual. Some stages may last for years, whereas a patient may pass through

Signs & Signals

HELPING PATIENTS COPE WITH ALZHEIMER DISEASE

Currently, there is no cure for Alzheimer disease. When caring for patients who have Alzheimer disease, remember that their feelings of anger and frustration are symptoms of their disease, not to be taken personally. Keep the following tips in mind when caring for patients with Alzheimer disease:

- Treat patients with compassion and patience.
- Speak calmly and without sounding condescending.
- Never argue with the patient, even if the patient blames you for something he forgot.
- Reintroduce yourself at each appointment. The patient may not remember you from his last visit.
- Explain common procedures as if the patient is unfamiliar with them.
- Approach the patient quietly and professionally in a gentle manner. Remind the patient who you are and what you're going to be doing.
- Provide the patient, family members, and any caregivers with information on local support groups for Alzheimer disease.

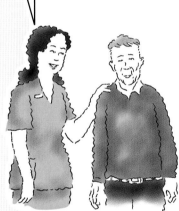

Never argue with patients who have Alzheimer disease. Instead, speak in a calm voice and use soothing therapeutic touch.

other stages rapidly. As a patient's disease progresses, you'll notice less responsiveness and mental agility. In the latter stages of the disease, patients are unaware of their disease and how it affects those around them.

Other Common Diseases

Several other diseases are commonly recognized among older adults, such as heart disease, pneumonia, and stroke. It's essential to be aware of the risks for these common diseases in geriatric patients. See the table on page 133 to become familiar with the warning signs and symptoms related to each disease.

Other Common Diseases in Older Adults			
Disease	**What Is It?**	**Who Is at Risk?**	**What Are the Signs and Symptoms?**
Heart disease	abnormality of the heart (or of the blood vessels supplying the heart with blood and oxygen) that impairs its normal functioning	older adults; especially smokers and the obese	angina (discomfort, heaviness, pressure, aching, burning, fullness, squeezing, or a painful feeling in the chest) shortness of breath palpitations or irregular heartbeat faster heartbeat weakness or dizziness nausea sweating myocardial infarction (heart attack)
Chronic obstructive pulmonary disease (COPD)	the combination of chronic bronchitis and emphysema	long-term smokers	shortness of breath chronic cough mucus production wheezing
Pneumonia	bacterial or viral infection in the alveoli (tiny sacs that are the site of gas exchange in the lungs)	older adults, because their immune systems are weaker	fever cough chills dyspnea (shortness of breath)
Stroke	a cardiovascular disease that affects the arteries leading to and within the brain	older adults, because they often suffer blood clots and vessel bursts, causing an obstruction of oxygen and nutrients to the brain	numbness or weakness in the face, arm, or leg, especially on one side of the body sudden confusion; trouble speaking or understanding sudden trouble seeing from one or both eyes sudden trouble walking; dizziness; loss of balance or coordination sudden, severe headache with no known cause
Type 2 diabetes	a disease in which the body doesn't produce or properly use insulin	individuals who are genetically predisposed to the disease; individuals who are obese; individuals who suffer from diabetes as a complication of another condition (such as heart disease)	blood glucose levels that are higher than normal increased thirst and frequent urination weight fluctuations blurred vision slow-healing sores or frequent infections nerve damage red, swollen, tender gums

ELDER ABUSE AND NEGLECT

Older adults are in a vulnerable state, especially when they're dependent on others for care and assistance. They have specific needs that require special attention from caregivers. Unfortunately, older adults are sometimes subject to abuse and mistreatment at the hands of the very people who are supposed to be helping them.

As a health care professional, it's your duty to protect older adult patients' well-being. One way you can do this is by knowing who is at risk for abuse, why it happens, and the warning signs that tell you something is wrong.

Risk Factors

The following are common risk factors for elder abuse.

- multiple chronic illnesses that stress the family's physical, emotional, and financial resources
- senile dementia that overrides reasoning abilities
- bladder or bowel incontinence
- age-related sleep disorders that disturb the caregiver's rest
- total dependence upon the caregiver to meet the patient's basic needs

Family members and spouses may be guilty of abuse or neglect, whether it's intentional or not. A caregiver may feel angry or unable to cope with the responsibility of providing care for the older adult patient and may unfairly take his feelings out on the patient.

Forms of Abuse and Neglect

Elder abuse and neglect can take different forms, including:

- passive neglect (when a patient's care is neglected unintentionally), often a result of the caregiver's ignorance regarding the patient's needs or due to the caregiver's inability to meet these needs
- active neglect, such as overmedicating the patient to render him passive and easier to care for
- psychological abuse, including threats, name-calling and put-downs, isolation, and withholding basic needs (such as nutrition)
- financial abuse, such as embezzling, squandering, or outright stealing money from the patient
- physical abuse, including smaller forms such as pinching and slapping, as well as life-threatening injuries
- sexual abuse

Warning Signs

If you suspect elder abuse or neglect, you are ethically and legally responsible to report your suspicion to the physician, who will contact the proper authorities. The signs of elder abuse include:

- wounds or markings of suspicious or unexplained origin
- wrist or ankle abrasions or bruising
- large pressure ulcers
- poor hygiene and nutrition
- dehydration not caused by a medical condition
- untreated injuries or medical conditions
- moodiness, agitation, apathy, or loss of will in the patient

Educating Family Members and Caregivers

As a medical assistant, you can help prevent elder abuse and neglect by educating family members and caregivers about the patient's condition. Ask family members if they need outside assistance and, if so, help them find it. Offer your support and answer any questions they have regarding the patient's condition and how they should care for her. Of course, if family members or caregivers ask any questions that you aren't qualified to answer, be sure to relate these questions to the physician. By educating family members and caregivers properly, you can help decrease the

Ask The Professional CROSSING THE LINE

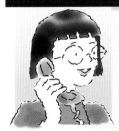

Q: *What should I do if I suspect a patient is being abused by a family member or caregiver?*

A: Sometimes, you may notice obvious physical signs of abuse, such as bruises on the body. But other times, the warning signs of abuse are more subtle. For example, a dominant family member may not allow the patient to talk for himself, or may seem impatient when the patient is slow or is taking a longer time to complete a task. If you suspect that one of your patients is being abused by a caregiver, promptly report your concerns to the physician or supervisor. The physician or supervisor will tell you what to do next, or she may decide to handle this situation herself. Either way, it's important that you report your concerns so the appropriate actions can be taken.

likelihood of elder abuse occurring. Educating the family members of older adult patients can also help them make informed decisions concerning the type and level of assistance needed.

> If the caregiver is having difficulty coping, he may benefit from professional help. Sometimes, just talking about the problem can make someone feel better!

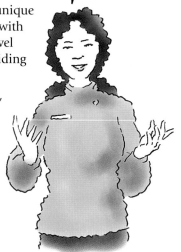

Caring for Children

Caring for children is a task that presents its own unique challenges for the medical staff. How you interact with and respond to children often depends on their level of maturity and stage of development. When providing care to children:

- keep in mind the child's development, growth, and maturity level
- explain procedures to the child on an age-appropriate level and gauge your responses to meet the child's emotional and mental needs
- develop new communication techniques
- recognize signs of abuse and neglect

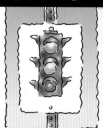

Signs & Signals — TIPS ON CARING FOR CHILDREN

Keep the following information in mind when caring for children.

- Children have active imaginations and are highly sensitive to the things happening around them. Everything seems louder, brighter, more painful, scarier, and so on.
- Children often respond by either verbalizing their fears or acting out (i.e., screaming, crying, squirming away).
- Children's concerns may be disproportionate to the actual threat of pain or danger. However, these fears and concerns are very real to the child and deserve validation from you.
- Parents and guardians are a source of support for children. Encourage them to stay in the examination room during procedures involving young children.

CHILD DEVELOPMENT

Understanding a child's psychological needs and development helps you provide effective, age-appropriate care. Here are some guidelines to follow when interacting with children of various age groups.

- *Infant (0–12 months old)*. The baby seeks to trust you. Use a soft, reassuring voice and gentle touch. Inform parents and guardians about the dangers of a high fever, vomiting, diarrhea, and the failure to nurse or take a bottle.
- *Toddler (13 months–3 years old)*. The child seeks independence. Expect resistance, and use a firm and direct approach. Ignore negative behavior and reward the positive. The child may try to squirm away, so take actions to protect his safety.
- *Preschooler (4–5 years old)*. The child uses his initiative. Encourage him to express how he's feeling and explain procedures to him in a way he can understand.
- *School-aged child (6–11 years old)*. The child is becoming industrious. Involve him in decision making and care. Encourage and support his questions.
- *Adolescent (12–18 years old)*. The adolescent is struggling with issues of identity and may resist authority figures. Discuss procedures so the adolescent can understand and avoid "talking down" to the patient. Patient education at this stage of development should include information on smoking, alcohol use, and perhaps birth control and STDs.

COMMUNICATING WITH CHILDREN

Levels of comprehension and maturity vary greatly from child to child. In general, the following behaviors will help you communicate with children.

- Get down to their level. Children respond to face-to-face communication at eye level; it creates a sense of equality.

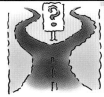

Fork in the Road   PROVIDING AGE-APPROPRIATE CARE

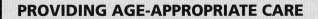

On the next page, match each age group in the first column with the medical assistant's correct behavior from the second column. Then, in one to two sentences, explain why each behavior is correct in terms of the child's stage of development.

1. infant (0–12 months)	a. Restrain the child to maintain safety during procedures.
2. toddler (13 months–3 years)	b. Encourage the child to speak his feelings.
3. preschooler (4–5 years)	c. Keep the parent in the child's view and use a soft, soothing voice.
4. school-aged child (6–11 years)	d. Make sure patient education includes information about smoking and alcohol use.
5. adolescent (12–18 years)	e. Involve the child in decision making.

- Keep your voice low-pitched and gentle.
- Make slow movements. Let a child know if you're about to touch him.
- Rephrase or simplify your questions until you're sure the child has understood them.
- Be prepared for the child to regress to former stages of development when under stress. For example, a child can regress to sucking his thumb when receiving an injection.
- Incorporate play creatively.
- Allow the child to express fear or cry.

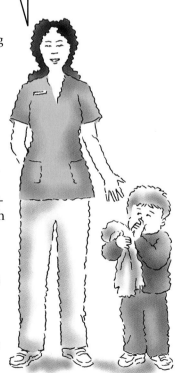

Children can revert to previous stages of development when under stress.

RECOGNIZING CHILD ABUSE AND NEGLECT

The signs of child abuse and neglect are often detectable when we communicate with children. A child may seem fearful or unwilling to discuss certain subjects with you. He may look at his parent uneasily before responding to questions, such as "How did you hurt yourself here?" It's important to consider a child's behavior when determining whether further action should be taken.

Child abuse and neglect compromise a child's social, emotional, and physical well-being. Although child abuse isn't always discussed openly, it is quite common in our society. Abuse is thought to be the second most common cause of death in children under the age of five years old. If abuse persists, a child can be physically or emotionally damaged for the rest of her life. This is why it's so important to be aware of the warning signs of abuse when interacting with children. If you recognize any of the common signs or symptoms of neglect, report your concerns to the physician immediately.

Signs of Abuse

Some of the more obvious signs of child abuse include the following:

- reports of physical or sexual abuse by the child
- previous reports of abuse or neglect within the family along with current signs
- conflicting stories about the "accident" or injury from the parent or caregiver and the child
- injuries inconsistent with the story provided
- injuries blamed on siblings or someone other than the parent
- repeated emergency room visits for injuries
- fractures, burns, or bone injuries of a suspicious nature

Sometimes, a parent or child will go to great lengths to hide the abuse from others. These are several physical signs of abuse that aren't always apparent:

- dislocations
- nervous system trauma, particularly shaken baby syndrome
- internal injuries, particularly to the abdominal area

Abused or neglected children will often display behaviors that don't match up with their level of age-appropriate development. The following behaviors can sometimes be an indication of abuse:

- too-willing compliance, or being overeager to please
- passive avoidance, such as refusing to make eye contact or turning away the body
- extremely aggressive, demanding, and rage-filled behavior, such as screaming, biting, or kicking
- role reversal ("parenting the parent"), including making excuses for a parent's poor behavior or inattention
- developmental delay (the child may be using energy needed for physical growth to defend himself against the abuse)

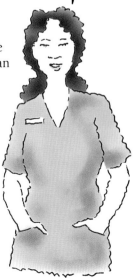

If you suspect child abuse or neglect, be sure to report your concerns to the physician. The physician is required by law to report suspected child abuse.

Signs of Neglect

The signs of neglect aren't always as noticeable as the signs of abuse. Neglect can often be hidden for a long period of time. In general, here are some signs of child neglect:

- malnutrition
- poor growth pattern
- poor hygiene
- extreme dental disorders
- unattended medical needs

Keep in mind that socioeconomic factors can play a part in a child's appearance and don't necessarily indicate neglect. For example, a parent may not be able to afford braces. If you ever suspect neglect, even if you are unsure, explain your concerns to the physician.

Adapting Teaching Material to the Patient

Educating patients about their own health is an often over-looked part of being a medical professional. Providing patients with the right educational materials and information is like providing them with the proper tools they need to change a tire. If they get a flat, they'll know how to change the tire on their own. If you teach patients about their own health care, they'll be less likely to return to you with the same ailments, and will feel that they have a hand in their own health care decisions.

To provide effective patient education, you must adjust your teaching methods to meet each patient's needs. If you make an effort to explain information and procedures in a way the patient can understand, he will be more likely to follow your advice at home. He will also feel that you are genuinely concerned about his overall health. Patients who can require specific teaching techniques include:

- children
- geriatric patients
- patients with illnesses
- non–English-speaking patients
- patients with physical impairments

CHILDREN

Children require different teaching strategies from you. Here are some ways you can help children listen to and understand the information you provide.

- Encourage the child to be part of the teaching process. For example, you might explain to a seven-year-old patient how to assemble an asthma nebulizer. Then, allow the child to assemble it by himself.
- Speak directly to the child.
- Avoid using confusing medical terms.
- Avoid using baby language.
- Teach only age-appropriate information.
- Discuss with parents their feelings concerning what the child should or should not know about his illness.
- Demonstrate procedures on stuffed animals or dolls first.
- Use pictures or flashcards when appropriate to explain a procedure.

Safety education is a prime teaching focus for young children and their parents. The Injury Prevention Program (TIPP) was developed by the American Academy of Pediatrics Committee on Injury, Violence, and Poison Prevention. The program provides age-appropriate safety education tips for children and their parents, such as the following.

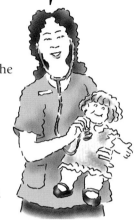

> Medical equipment can seem scary to young children. Examine the child's favorite doll first so she knows it's safe!

- *Birth to 6 months.* Stress the importance of proper car safety seat installation and usage. The safety seat should be installed according to the manufacturer's instructions and the owner's manual of the car. Children should be placed in safety seats every time they ride in the car.

> If a child eats or drinks a poisonous substance, parents should call the Poison Help Line immediately: 1-800-222-1222. Encourage parents to keep this number by the phone in case of emergency.

- *6 to 12 months.* Once children begin crawling and walking, parents should install gates on stairways and doors. Any windows above the first floor should be equipped with window guards to prevent falls. Inform parents that baby walkers can cause falls and therefore should *not* be used.
- *1 to 2 years.* Caution parents about burn prevention. Children who are just learning to walk will use any stationary object to steady themselves, including oven doors and heating units. When parents are preparing hot foods in the kitchen, the safest place for the child is in a high chair, playpen, or crib.
- *2 to 4 years.* Remind parents to place safety caps on medications and cleaning solutions. These substances should also be kept out of the child's reach.

- *5 years.* Educate parents and children about water safety. Children should never be allowed to swim unsupervised.

- *6 years.* Teach children about safety precautions to take when they play outside. Children should wear helmets when they're riding their bikes and they should never cross the street without an adult.

- *8 years.* Discuss car safety with parents and children. Children must use a booster seat until they can wear a lap and shoulder belt properly. Most states specify an age or height requirement. Check your state's laws so you can keep parents informed.

- *10 years.* For children who play sports, stress the importance of wearing protective gear, such as helmets, shin guards, and pads.

For additional safety tips, visit the American Academy of Pediatrics website: www.aap.org.

GERIATRIC PATIENTS

When providing education to geriatric patients, follow the same guidelines you learned for providing care to older adult patients, such as the following.

- Include the patient's family members in patient education, especially if they are the caregivers.

- Take the time to listen to each patient's questions and concerns. Avoid rushing the patient, and give him your full attention.

- Whether you're educating a patient about a particular medical condition or about the physician's prescribed treatment plan, use layman's terms and avoid using medical jargon.

- Provide patients with written instructions to take home as a reminder.

- Encourage patients to take an active role in their own daily health regimen. Have them apply bandages or ointments by themselves, and teach them how doing these things can improve their health.

A common topic you may teach older adult patients is self-medication. Educating geriatric patients about this topic can sometimes be a challenge, especially in patients with cognitive impairments (such as dementia). For example, a patient may be taking several different medications for various disorders. At the same time, the patient's body is coping with the added stress of illness, disease, and injury from decreased functioning of the body's systems. So, if a patient is taking more medications, he may be more likely to forget to take them. It's your responsibility to ensure that the patient adheres to the physician's prescribed medication regimen.

Here are some tips to follow when educating older adults about medication.

- Explain all the side effects and precautions to take with the prescribed medicines in a way that the patient can understand. Inform the patient when he shouldn't mix certain foods, beverages, and medications together.
- Explain the proper dosage and how to measure it.
- Write out a schedule for the patient and help the patient find ways of remembering it. For example, a patient may find it helpful to purchase a plastic pill holder with the days of the week and/or times of day inscribed on the front.
- Tell the patient to take the most important medication first.
- Advise the patient to take medication while sitting or standing straight, not reclining. Remind the patient to take one pill at a time with lots of water. If the medication is difficult to swallow, have the patient try placing the pill on the back of the tongue and drinking water through a straw.
- A patient with impaired eyesight can ask the pharmacist for enlarged labels. This decreases the chances of a medication error. Tell the patient that he can also request a non–child-proof container if there are no children in the home.
- Explain that the full dose of medication must be taken until it's gone (or according to the physician's instructions).
- Explain that no medication should be taken by another person or saved for another illness.

PATIENTS WITH ILLNESSES

A patient with recurring or frequent illnesses may find it difficult to focus on the new knowledge you're giving him. When educating a patient who is suffering from an illness, make sure the patient is comfortable first. Have him sit in a soft chair, and limit outside distractions. Give the patient enough time to process the information before responding to any questions or concerns he has. It's also helpful to provide written materials that the patient can take home and read again when he may be feeling better or more focused.

NON–ENGLISH-SPEAKING PATIENTS

Non–English-speaking patients may be willing to learn, but they'll require additional assistance to understand your message fully. As you learned earlier in this chapter, there are several ways to improve your communication with non–English-speaking patients.

For example, consider using a translator when educating patients about their health care. If someone in the medical office can act as an interpreter, then ask her to assist you with these patients. If a translator is not available, refer to a book of common phrases in the patient's native language.

When educating non–English-speaking patients, it's also important to provide written materials and visual aids. The medical office should be supplied with pamphlets and other educational materials written in languages common to the community. Pictures and visual aids can help you further explain procedures or treatments to a patient when language skills are limited.

PATIENTS WITH PHYSICAL IMPAIRMENTS

Physical impairments can slow down the learning process. For example, a patient with severe arthritis may have trouble performing certain psychomotor skills, like changing bandages on a wound. An occupational therapist is the best resource for helping you educate patients with physical impairments.

OTHER PATIENTS

Other factors can hinder your ability to educate patients effectively. For example, patients from certain cultural or religious backgrounds may not be willing to learn and incorporate new health care knowledge into their lifestyles. Patients with financial troubles may not be ready to focus on learning new skills or information. In these situations, it's important that you assess the patient's commitment to learning and help the patient remove any obstacles that might prevent learning.

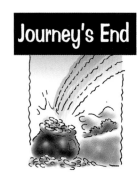

Journey's End

- Cultural diversity refers to the differences that individuals and groups bring to a culture. As a medical assistant, you should understand how cultural beliefs, attitudes, and practices affect the health care needs of each patient.

- Certain cultural beliefs and customs, such as those regarding reactions to pain, can affect the health care that a person receives. Because some cultures discourage the open expression of pain, it's important to pay attention to each patient's body language.

- Provide culturally sensitive care to patients by being aware of your own cultural background and how it affects your health care.
- When assisting patients with special needs, understand and be sensitive to the degree to which they're disabled. Then, adjust your care accordingly. Focus on patients' abilities and work with them to provide compassionate care.
- When caring for geriatric patients, be aware of issues such as decreased mobility, the effects of aging on the body, concurrent illnesses, and polypharmacy. Treat each patient as an individual with unique abilities and needs.
- You can develop trusting relationships with young children and their parents by encouraging parental involvement and providing age-appropriate care to children.
- Some patients, such as children, non–English-speaking patients, and patients with physical impairments, have specific needs when it comes to patient education. Be sure to adapt your teaching plan appropriately for each patient you instruct.

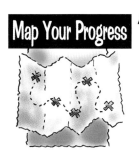

Map Your Progress

Answer the following multiple-choice questions.

1. What is *cultural diversity?*
   a. the differences between people
   b. the similarities between people
   c. the way culture affects health care
   d. the way special needs affect health care

2. Which of the following cultural elements affects patients' health care?
   a. genetic disposition to certain diseases or disorders
   b. cultural attitudes concerning pain and emotional expression
   c. cultural attitudes concerning modesty
   d. all of the above

3. Language barriers are:
   a. nonverbal forms of communication, such as facial expressions and body language.
   b. hearing impairments.
   c. cultural differences concerning personal space.
   d. "roadblocks" to effective communication.

4. The belief that one's own ideas, beliefs, and practices are superior and preferable to others is:
   a. ethnocentrism.
   b. bias.
   c. stereotyping.
   d. discrimination.

5. Which of the following is an example of a *developmental disability?*
   a. type 2 diabetes
   b. Alzheimer disease
   c. Down syndrome
   d. bipolar disorder

6. Suppose a patient arrives for his appointment and tells you, "I think I have the flu." What should you do to help control the spread of infection?
   a. Have him wait for the physician in a private examination room instead of in the waiting room.
   b. Tell the patient to go home, rest, and drink plenty of fluids. Advise him to call the physician if his symptoms don't improve.
   c. Ask the patient to wear appropriate PPE, such as a mask and disposable gloves, while he's in the office.
   d. none of the above

7. Why is it important to educate caregivers of older adults?
   a. to provide information about Parkinson disease
   b. to take up time after examinations while the patient gets dressed
   c. to prevent elder abuse
   d. to decrease risk of suicide

8. Which of the following is *not* a sign of child abuse?
   a. suspicious bruises or scars
   b. poor nutrition
   c. lack of exercise
   d. overeagerness to please

9. Polypharmacy is:
   a. the use of two pharmacies simultaneously.
   b. the use of multiple medications simultaneously.
   c. the dosage prescribed.
   d. the potential side effects of a medication.

10. Which of the following techniques should you use to help a child listen to and understand the information you provide?
    a. Be friendly and use baby language.
    b. Speak directly to the parent, instead of to the child.
    c. Use large, clear print in written instructions.
    d. Demonstrate procedures on stuffed animals or dolls first.

Chapter 5

MAKING THE MOST OF YOUR EXTERNSHIP EXPERIENCE

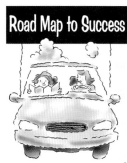

Road Map to Success

- Explain the value of an externship in helping you become a successful medical assistant

- Identify the different types of externship facilities

- List the purpose and goals of the externship experience

- Explain the importance of applying the good habits you've learned in the classroom to your externship experience

- Identify ways in which you can prepare yourself for your externship mentally, physically, and professionally

- Explain how you can make a good first impression on your supervisors at the externship site

- Identify key tasks and expectations involved in an externship program

- Explain how you can protect patient rights under HIPAA during your externship

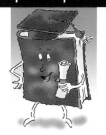

Chapter Competencies

- Project a positive attitude (ABHES 1.a.)

- Adapt to change (ABHES 1.f.)

- Be a "team player" (ABHES 1.c.)

- Maintain confidentiality at all times (ABHES 1.b.)

- Identify and respond to issues of confidentiality (CAAHEP 3.c.2.a.)

The externship is an important part of your journey to professionalism. This chapter will provide tips for making your externship a successful experience. You'll also learn the following information:

- the types of externship facilities and the benefits of the externship
- how to prepare mentally, physically, and professionally for the externship
- how to have a successful interview and make a good first impression
- how a medical office operates
- the tasks involved in the externship
- how to interact with coworkers and care for patients
- how to abide by HIPAA policies

The Externship: A Window of Opportunity

When you learn something new, you gather knowledge and experience about the subject. Knowledge is the information you need to master to reach your goals. Experience is important because it helps you test your knowledge.

As a medical assistant in training, you'll need to practice your skills before successfully completing the program. An **externship** is a period of time during which you work in a medical office while you're still a student. The externship occurs during your final term in school, usually after you've passed all other required courses in the program. It varies in length from 60 to 240 hours, depending on your school's curriculum and the medical site where you'll be working. Although you won't be paid for the work you do during the externship, you'll receive credit toward your degree or certificate plan. Here are the basic steps you'll follow to arrange your externship.

1. First, you'll select or be assigned to a particular externship site. Most medical assisting programs have a **clinical coordinator** who matches students to appropriate sites chosen by the school.

2. Next, you'll meet with your school's clinical coordinator to discuss important details about the medical facility where you'll be conducting your externship.

3. Finally, you'll be assigned a **preceptor** who will work with you at the externship site. Depending on the site, your preceptor may be a graduate medical assistant, licensed practical nurse, or registered nurse.

Under the supervision of your preceptor or supervisor, you'll have the opportunity to gain hands-on experience. Your preceptor will assist you as you apply the theories and procedures you have learned in the classroom. You'll also discover areas of medicine in which you might be particularly interested.

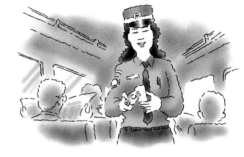

All aboard the Externship Express! Take a journey to discover all that awaits you in the medical assisting field.

TYPES OF EXTERNSHIP FACILITIES

The health care industry includes a wide variety of specialty offices and clinics to treat the needs of many different kinds of patients. You may complete your externship in a family or general practice facility, where you'll practice a wide range of skills. Or you may complete your externship at a specialty practice, where you'll learn the specific skills used in that particular field of medicine. Both general and specialty practices offer the experience you'll need to gain entry into the world of medical assisting.

General and Family Practices

Physicians who work in general or family practices are often referred to as primary care providers or internists. General practitioners treat a wide variety of complaints and illnesses. Family practitioners also see patients who have various illnesses; however, their patients will usually range in age from newborn to adult, whereas a general practitioner may only treat adult patients.

The advantage of completing your externship in a general or family practice is the exposure you'll have to all types of procedures performed by medical assistants, which will widen your scope of skills and abilities. If, however, you're interested in eventually working in a particular specialty, then you may not have a chance to experience the procedures and skills that are specific to that specialty. In that case, you may want to pursue your externship at a specialty practice instead.

Specialty Practices

Specialists are physicians who focus on a particular field of medicine. The following are several examples of specialists who employ medical assistants.

- Pediatricians provide medical care to children and treat childhood disorders.

- Dermatologists diagnose and treat skin disorders.
- Orthopedists diagnose and treat disorders of the musculo-skeletal system.
- Obstetricians limit their practices to care and treatment for pregnancy, the postpartum ("after birth") period, and fertility issues.
- Cardiologists diagnose and treat disorders of the heart, arteries, and veins.
- Podiatrists diagnose and treat disorders of the feet.

Because specialty practices focus on very specific areas of care, you may not experience the broad range of procedures and tasks that you would at a family practitioner's office. For example, staff members in an obstetrics office usually don't perform electrocardiograms, and staff members in an orthopedic office don't perform pregnancy tests.

However, conducting your externship in a specialty practice has its advantages, too. By working in a specialty facility, you'll gain experience in observing and performing the special examinations and procedures that you might not observe in a general practice setting. Conducting your externship in a specialty practice may make you a more desirable candidate when you are seeking job opportunities, because other medical assistants may not have had the same experience.

MENTORSHIP

If you went to summer camp as a child, then there's a good chance you know a thing or two about the "Big Brother" and "Big Sister" programs. Your big brother or sister acted as a **mentor,** guiding you through camp life and helping you out when you needed it. Maybe you were a mentor yourself and knew how to provide a safety net for other people. Now you're an adult, and your career goal is clear: to become a professional medical assistant. But that doesn't mean you have to go it alone.

Your preceptor will act as your mentor throughout the externship program. Often, preceptors are medical assistants who have graduated from a medical assisting program and who have experienced a similar externship program. Preceptors work with externship students similar to the way instructors work with students in the classroom. They can provide you with valuable advice and insights about medical assisting.

Most schools have externship sites that they have used for years. Schools are careful to choose externship sites with preceptors who are willing to work with you and help you feel comfortable in the medical setting. Until now, you've only practiced your skills inside the classroom with fellow students, so you may be nervous about leaving the comfort of a controlled setting. Preceptors understand what you're going through because they've been through it themselves. They know what it takes to ease you into the transition from classroom to medical office. Preceptors are a fountain of knowledge and resources, so never be afraid to ask for help. That's what they're there for!

> Your preceptor helps cushion the experience; he will catch you if you fall!

HANDS-ON EXPERIENCE

Leaving the classroom and actually putting your skills to use in a medical office can be extremely rewarding, even if it seems nerve-wracking at first. Take the opportunity to absorb as much as possible from your externship experience. Think of the medical facility as your new classroom and the staff as its teachers. The medical staff is responsible for providing you with the

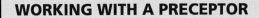

Travelog   WORKING WITH A PRECEPTOR

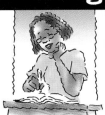

As a medical assisting student with no experience in a medical setting, I was nervous about completing the externship. I'd never practiced my skills outside the classroom or even seen some of the equipment I would be using, except in textbooks. I felt relieved when I learned that a preceptor would be working closely with us. The preceptor was so helpful! She put me at ease by explaining procedures and techniques in detail and answering my questions. Once, during training, I was asked to take an infant's blood pressure. I was so afraid of hurting him! My preceptor showed me where to place the blood pressure cuff and how to read it. I felt much better knowing that I could ask for help if I needed it. Her assistance was similar to that of the classroom instructor, which helped make my transition from the classroom to the medical office that much smoother. My preceptor was an invaluable help to me during my externship experience!

opportunities for training. The staff will also help you become familiar with office policies and procedures.

At some sites, students are only allowed to observe more complex procedures such as administering injections, but they're often given permission to perform some basic or routine procedures such as taking vital signs. Even if you aren't allowed to perform every procedure, you'll still have the opportunity to observe, take notes, and ask questions. You'll also get a feel for what it's like to work with patients and coworkers. The hands-on experience you gain during the externship will be useful to you later when you enter the medical assisting field.

Using Your Technical Skills

The first step toward engaging in any kind of hands-on experience is taking the initiative to make it happen. During the externship, learning isn't just about theory and knowledge. You'll also have the opportunity to practice the technical skills you observed in the classroom.

For some skills, you may have simply watched the instructor perform a demonstration or viewed a video of the procedure. It's understandable that you might still be unsure how to perform these procedures or tasks. Here are some tips to keep in mind when learning how to use and perfect your technical skills at the externship site.

- Take every opportunity to observe other health care professionals performing basic medical procedures. For example, you might observe a nurse drawing a blood specimen. Pay attention to the technique he uses and make mental notes of changes you can make to improve your own technical skills.

- If you're unsure how to operate a piece of medical equipment or perform a particular procedure, ask questions! Your preceptor and the other health care professionals in the office are there to help you learn.

- Refer to flash cards or pocket guides to medical assisting containing step-by-step instructions for each procedure. These reminders will help you perform each step correctly and in the proper order.

- If you're allowed to perform procedures involving needles or syringes at the externship site, do so *only* under the direct supervision of a qualified professional. If performed incorrectly, these procedures can endanger patients' safety.

- Remember that practice makes perfect. The more you practice a skill in the medical office, the more confident you'll feel, and the easier that skill will become.

You'll be judged on your ability to perform procedures by the same standard of care as is expected of an entry-level medical assistant. Your preceptor is there to help you, but it's best to come to your externship prepared. Practicing skills inside the classroom or skills laboratory first will start you off on the right foot.

> The externship gives you opportunities to practice your technical skills on actual patients. Your preceptor or another qualified health care professional will supervise the procedures you perform.

Enhancing Your "Soft Skills"

The externship will also allow you to practice and enhance your "soft skills," such as communication and customer service. "Soft skills" are sometimes referred to as "people skills."

During the externship, you'll get the opportunity to work with actual patients. Doing so will help you learn how to identify and accommodate patients' different needs. By practicing these skills, you'll also learn how to provide high-quality care. For example, elderly patients with mobility difficulties may require your assistance when sitting, standing, or undressing for exams and procedures. Helping patients with these tasks requires patience and sensitivity on your part, and you'll learn how incorporating these skills into your routine can help patients feel more comfortable.

Here are some tips to help you improve your soft skills while you're working with patients.

- Be aware of your body language. Smiling while relaxing your arms and maintaining good posture shows the patient that you're friendly and ready to help.

- Be aware of patients' body language. Frowning, crossed arms, or clenched fists are all indications that the patient is uncomfortable or in pain. Recognize these signs and ask the patient, "How can I help you?"

- Think about your own medical experiences. Have you encountered health care professionals who were extremely helpful and made you feel comfortable? What did they do? How did their actions make you feel?

> Ms. Young, let me show you to an examination room where you might be more comfortable waiting for the physician.

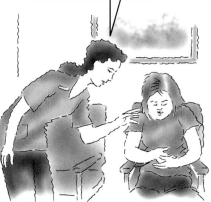

Consider how your personal experiences can help you provide better care.

- Talk to the person, not the problem. Remember that patients are real people, and their lives are about more than their illnesses. Be respectful and caring in all your interactions with patients.

SKILLS ASSESSMENT

By the end of your classroom experience, you'll have memorized and studied textbooks, observed professionals, and asked lots of questions. You may have practiced your skills so much that you're now performing them in your sleep! But will you have reached the level of a professional medical assistant?

The skills assessment is another helpful part of the externship experience. It's a tool you can use to understand where your strengths and weaknesses lie, and how you can become a better medical assistant. Your abilities and skill level will be carefully considered by your medical assisting program's clinical coordinator, who will evaluate your progress during and after the completion of the externship. At the end of your externship, you'll also complete a self-evaluation form.

Making the Grade

After you've begun your externship, your school's clinical coordinator will visit or call frequently to follow your progress. The clinical coordinator acts as a liaison between you and the externship site. If either you or the site has concerns during your externship, the clinical coordinator will mediate to help resolve any conflicts or problems that may arise.

Whereas your preceptor works with you daily as a mentor, the clinical coordinator will periodically evaluate what you've learned. The coordinator will most likely use an evaluation form that includes detailed areas to be graded. These are similar to grades you'd receive on a test or examination. Your clinical coordinator will use these evaluations to determine whether you're ready to enter the field of medical assisting or if you need additional training. You can keep track of your progress by having frequent conferences with your clinical coordinator.

Taking a Good Look at Yourself

You will complete a self-evaluation form after your externship has ended. Completing this form will help you identify your professional strengths and weaknesses. It will also help

Road Rules   EXTERNSHIP BENEFITS

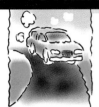

It's important to keep in mind all of the benefits of the externship. These benefits can motivate you to keep working hard toward your goal of becoming a professional medical assistant. Remember that the externship will:

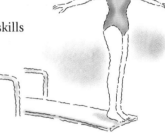

The experience you'll gain during the externship will help you "dive in" to your medical assisting career!

- provide you with hands-on experience working in a medical office
- teach you how to work well with patients and coworkers in a medical setting
- give you the opportunity to practice your skills and learn from trained professionals
- provide you with constructive criticism so you can improve and refine your skills
- possibly help you determine your interest in a particular medical specialty

you determine which technical or other skills you still need to develop or enhance. Be honest with yourself as you evaluate your performance. Take the time to list the things you performed well and are proud of, as well as the things you could improve upon.

Preparing for Your Externship

Preparing for your externship isn't just about having successfully completed all the classroom requirements. It's about feeling mentally and physically prepared to face challenges and learn from the experience. To have a satisfying externship experience, you'll likely need to:

- find ways of reducing anxiety and stress
- get proper rest and nutrition
- learn to manage your time wisely
- learn how to prioritize
- seek help from family and friends

MENTAL PREPARATION

You've studied hard, you've practiced your skills, and now you're about to put your knowledge to the test in a real medical office. By now, you may feel like an old pro in the classroom, so you may be wondering, "Why do I feel so anxious now?" The externship is like any new experience; to do your best, you need to feel mentally prepared! You can't always predict what will come your way, but there are some tips and strategies you can master to curb your anxiety and keep a level head.

Avoiding Anxiety

It's normal to feel nervous the first time you talk with a patient or perform technical skills, such as taking a patient's blood pressure or giving an injection. A little anxiety probably won't affect your clinical performance, but too much anxiety can interfere with your ability to practice and learn. If you begin to feel the anxiety getting the better of you, take a minute to consider the following suggestions:

- Take a time-out. If you're feeling overwhelmed by the pressure to perform, take a step back to gather your thoughts. If possible, take a walk or get a drink of water. Return to the situation when you feel relaxed and ready to proceed.

- Be flexible. Unexpected tasks and situations will inevitably arise. It isn't always possible to plan for everything. Learning how to "go with the flow" and respond to problems as they arise will decrease your anxiety.

- Ask for help. It's better to ask your preceptor or another staff member for assistance than to perform a procedure or task incorrectly.

- Use available resources. Review your flash cards or your pocket guide to medical assisting if you're having trouble remembering something.

- Seek out new information. Don't expect others to come to you. Seeking out the answers to your questions shows courage and initiative and can alleviate the anxiety you feel about not knowing the answers.

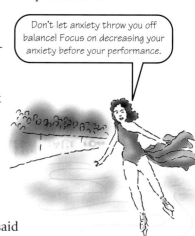

Don't let anxiety throw you off balance! Focus on decreasing your anxiety before your performance.

Reducing Stress

Reducing stress is like losing weight—easier said than done! But there are a number of techniques you can choose from that can reduce the stress you experience during your externship. Take a look at these tips and see which ones will work for you.

- Eliminate stressors. Many things cause stress, but the buildup of chronically stressful tasks and events can cause real health problems. So, find ways of avoiding them. For example, you might take a different route to work to avoid traffic.
- Learn how to relax. Find a comfortable position, breathe deeply, and just do nothing. Clear your mind and focus on positive thoughts or affirmations, such as "I can do this."
- Get a massage. A good massage will relax your muscles and increase circulation, resulting in improved mental functioning. Massage also triggers the release of endorphins, the body's natural pain relievers.
- Exercise your mind. When you're feeling stressed, visualize yourself in a quiet, safe place. For example, see yourself in a forest. Experience the colors, the smells, and nature's beauty. Focus on the good feelings and sensations that the image gives you.
- Learn to meditate. Focus on an object to eliminate distractions in your mind. You may choose to focus on a repetitive sound, a peaceful image, or deep breathing exercises. Meditation will decrease worried thoughts.
- Practice yoga. Yoga combines mental, physical, and spiritual energies to promote health and wellness. The basic components of yoga include proper breathing, movement, and posture, all of which enhance your energy level.
- Take a walk. Walking increases blood flow to the brain, allowing you to think more clearly. Walking also gives you time to "decompress" and think about the day's activities.
- Exercise regularly. Regular exercise increases endorphins, the feel-good chemicals in your brain. Exercise also strengthens your body, increases your energy during the day, and helps you sleep better at night.
- Take a bubble bath. Fill a tub with warm water and let the day's troubles wash away.
- Learn Tai Chi. Tai Chi is a martial art and type of exercise that promotes health and longevity.

Learning how to deal with and let go of stress during your externship will help you later when you're working as a medical assistant. Pay attention to the ways in which your instructors, coworkers, and other experienced professionals handle stress. Ask them if they have any suggestions for you.

PHYSICAL PREPARATION

So you've reduced your anxiety and eliminated some of the stressors in your life. Your mind is clear and ready for action, but what about the rest of you? Your body demands just as much care and attention as your brain. Taking the time to prepare physically for your externship will lead to:

- increased efficiency and skillfulness
- better memory retention
- improved learning and mental activity

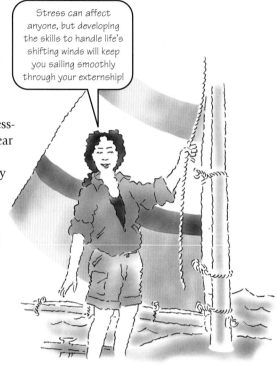

Stress can affect anyone, but developing the skills to handle life's shifting winds will keep you sailing smoothly through your externship!

Diet and Exercise

An important part of physical preparation is being mindful of your diet and exercise habits. Eating a healthy, balanced diet and getting enough exercise every day will give you the energy you need to meet the demands of your externship. Follow these healthful suggestions to keep your body in top shape.

- Remember that every little bit helps. Exercising a few times a week or even keeping up with a daily regimen of stretches in the morning can help lower stress, keep you alert, and help you feel good.

- Choose an activity you enjoy. Running several miles can burn a lot of calories, but if you don't enjoy it, then you're less likely to do it consistently.

- Reduce your caffeine intake. It may keep you awake, but caffeine also stimulates the sympathetic nervous system and produces tension and anxiety, making you more tired and stressed in the long run.

- Curb your sweet tooth. Avoid sugary foods, because they can lead to sudden increases and decreases in blood glucose, affecting your ability to concentrate and think clearly.

- Get your vitamins. During periods of stress, increasing your intake of fruits and vegetables (excellent sources of vitamins B and C and folic acid) will enhance your body's ability to cope with everyday stresses.

> Remember to eat breakfast—it gives you the fuel you need to start your day!

Proper Rest

Eating a healthy diet and exercising regularly aren't the only ways to increase your energy. During sleep, your body replenishes its energy sources, so you wake up feeling refreshed and ready to start the day. However, if you don't get enough sleep, you won't feel rested, and your ability to perform well and handle stress will be compromised. Follow these tips to get better shut-eye.

- Get at least eight hours of sleep every night. Lack of sleep will catch up with you, causing you to "crash" later in the day.

- Go to bed and wake up at the same time every day. This kind of routine will train your mind and body to stay on track.

- Avoid caffeine for several hours before bedtime. Try to relax and "wind down" before going to bed.

- Listen to your body. If you're feeling sleepy, then go to bed. Sometimes, it's more important to get that extra hour of sleep than to finish a small task.

Some people have difficulty falling or staying asleep. If this sounds like you, then you might consider consulting your physician to determine why you're having trouble sleeping and what you can do about it.

Vaccinations

Getting the appropriate vaccinations is another way that you're expected to prepare your body for the externship experience. Your medical assisting program is responsible for maintaining liability insurance for students during their externship. Because of this, students are generally required to provide proof of general immunizations and vaccination for hepatitis B. Students are allowed to provide proof by way of blood titer as well as documentation.

Required vaccinations include proof of MMR vaccination and chickenpox (disease or vaccination). Some facilities provide the hepatitis B vaccine for students. Most programs also require a:

- current physical examination
- serology profile (immunization record)
- tuberculin skin test

These requirements usually must be met before you are admitted to the externship program or before having direct contact with patients. Preparing for these requirements and meeting all deadlines will keep you on the right track toward completing your externship.

Other Factors

Keep in mind that some extern sites require drug screens and criminal background checks before beginning your work on site. It's important to comply with these procedures so that you may participate in the externship to the fullest of your ability.

PROFESSIONAL PREPARATION

You can also prepare for the externship by doing many of the same things that prepare you for your work in the classroom. The habits that work well for you as a student can also apply to the externship. They might include:

- managing your time
- establishing priorities
- asking for help

Time Management

The externship experience will make new demands on your time and energy. It's important to understand how much time to reserve for professional and personal activities so you can plan ahead. Managing your time wisely is an important skill that will also help you:

- decrease your stress and anxiety
- organize and complete your tasks so they meet all expectations
- balance your professional, personal, and social activities
- keep on track toward completing your externship and working in the medical field

Managing your time is like managing any other aspect of your life-it takes practice and dedication. It can be easy to procrastinate or find yourself preoccupied when you should be completing a task. Some people are very organized and decisive, whereas others are content to work on many tasks at once or allow themselves to get caught up in the flow of events as they unfold. Both styles can be effective, but it's important to understand how they influence the way you manage your time. Once you understand how much time to devote to certain tasks

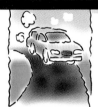

Road Rules   MANAGING YOUR TIME WISELY

Have you heard the old saying, "Time flies when you're having fun"? Well, it can be just as true when you're trying to juggle several tasks at once! Before you know it, half the day is gone and you haven't accomplished nearly as much as you had set out to do. Does this sound familiar? If so, here are some tips to help you manage your time wisely.

- Write things down on a personal calendar. A calendar will help you keep track of all of your obligations and important dates. It will also help you plan ahead.

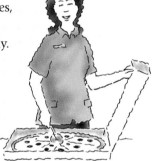

Manage your time by slicing large tasks into smaller ones.

- Avoid spending too much time on noncritical tasks. These tasks can become distracting, and before you know it, you've neglected the larger, more important tasks on your list.

- Avoid allowing large tasks to intimidate you. Break large tasks down into smaller, manageable ones, and you'll avoid the urge to procrastinate.

- All work and no play can stress you out quickly. Likewise, neglecting your externship duties in favor of personal pursuits will rob you of an enriching learning experience.

- Allow some breathing room in your schedule. Compulsively looking at the clock can stress you out even more than having too much to do.

and which tasks are the most important to you, you'll be better able to manage your time. But time management is also a life skill, so it's something you should always try to work on and improve.

Establishing Priorities

As a student, you are asked to manage many activities and obligations at the same time. Going to classes, studying and preparing for class, working, participating in sports or clubs, fulfilling family obligations, and exercising are just a few of the things that may be included on your to-do list. Trying to fit all those activities into one day can seem difficult enough. And now you're planning to add one more thing to that list: your externship. How are you going to complete all these tasks without becoming overly stressed? There are only so many hours in a day, so it's important that you establish priorities. Prioritizing means deciding which activities are the most and least important, and managing your time accordingly. Here are some useful tips to follow when prioritizing.

- Make a list of all the things you need to accomplish within a given time frame. For example, if you need to accomplish several tasks between the hours of 8:00 A.M. and 12:00 P.M., group those tasks together on your daily to-do list.
- Be realistic. Avoid scheduling too many tasks in one time period; it will just encourage you to procrastinate!
- Ask yourself, "Which of these tasks are the most important or urgent?" and, "Which tasks can be saved for later?" Complete the high-priority tasks first.
- Delegate a task or activity to someone else when possible. For example, when working on a group project, you shouldn't feel responsible for every task. Share the workload with others when you can.
- Be flexible. You may have to adjust your priorities if a new situation arises, such as a deadline change or family emergency.
- Simplify your life. Cut out activities and distractions that clutter your schedule. Don't be afraid to say "no" to some tasks or activities that are less important or beneficial for you.

Above all, remember: nobody's perfect! Avoid being too hard on yourself. Your externship isn't a race to the finish line, so pace yourself. You may not be able to complete every task, but if you set priorities, you'll know which tasks are most important and which you can save for another day.

Help from Family and Friends

Enlisting the support of your family and/or friends can be extremely important as you work your way through the externship process. Let your loved ones know when you'll be busy, and don't be afraid to ask for their help when you need it. Reaching out to others when you feel overwhelmed can lower your stress level and help you find solutions.

For example, if you have young children, you could ask a friend to babysit when you have another obligation to fulfill. Your loved ones will probably be happy to help you in any way they can. But if you're feeling unsure, have a sincere and hon-

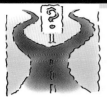

Fork in the Road   **KEEPING YOUR BALANCE**

Suppose your externship is taking a lot of your time and energy, and you're having a hard time balancing other life priorities. What should you do? In three to five sentences, list some suggestions for how you would handle the situation.

est talk with your family and friends, and let them know how you're feeling and how they can help. Decreasing the anxiety in your personal life will relieve some of the anxiety you may have about the externship.

DOWN TO THE LAST DETAIL

As you're well aware of by now, preparation is the key to having a successful externship experience. It's important to tie together any loose ends before you begin the externship. Here are some things to consider.

- *Transportation.* Will you have reliable transportation to and from the externship site every day? If you don't have a car, do you have access to public transportation? Can you arrange to carpool with someone else?

- *Child care services.* If you have young children, will they have a safe and reliable place to stay while you're at the externship site? Asking a friend or relative for help may be cost effective. Consider all your options.

- *Coverage.* Is there a backup system in place in case your child is sick, dismissed early, or if school is cancelled due to inclement weather? Form a backup plan and talk to your child about it.

- *Financial support.* Will you have financial coverage in case you have to miss some hours from work due to your externship? Do you have the full support of your boss and coworkers, and are they aware of this change in your schedule?

Beginning Your Externship

You've prepared for the externship like you would prepare for a test, and now the day to begin has finally arrived. You're ready to show everyone what you're made of. But beginning your externship is more than just learning a few basic procedures. It's about being prepared to do your best every single day. Beginning your externship will require that you:

- learn interview techniques
- make a good first impression
- dress professionally and manage your appearance
- maintain good attendance
- keep a positive attitude

THE INTERVIEW

Before beginning your externship, you may have an interview at the site with the physician and/or office manager. This interview is the first opportunity you'll have to make a good impression. So, treat this interview as if it were an actual job interview. What will you say? How will you represent yourself? Learning the proper protocol for interviews will let your supervisors know that you see the externship as a serious opportunity to learn and grow as a medical assistant in training.

The following are some general guidelines to help you have a successful interview.

- Practice the interview first with family members or friends. Have them ask you typical interview questions, and practice developing a relaxed demeanor.
- Rehearse what you might say in front of a mirror.
- Remember to be polite. Shake hands with the physician or office manager before and after the interview.
- Sell yourself. Be proud of your accomplishments, and don't be afraid to share them.
- Have a good grasp of your strengths and weaknesses. If the interviewer asks, explain what your weaknesses are and what you plan to do to improve your skills.

You'll learn additional interview tips in Chapter 6.

FIRST IMPRESSIONS

First impressions are lasting. When you meet someone new, you form an opinion of that person based on how he looks, behaves, and interacts with other people. It's important to make a good first impression on your preceptor, clinical coordinator, and supervising physician. Remember that these individuals will be evaluating your level of commitment and qualifications based on the externship site's standards, or criteria.

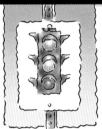

Signs & Signals — MAKING A GOOD FIRST IMPRESSION

Follow these tips to make an outstanding first impression:

- Smile and greet others warmly.
- Remember people's names and use them when communicating.
- Communicate your desire to help.
- Display "open" body language. Keep your arms uncrossed, make eye contact, and have a pleasant smile.
- Listen attentively and don't interrupt others who are speaking. Add a comment or ask questions when appropriate.
- Be sincere and honest.
- Speak clearly and thoughtfully.

GETTING TO KNOW YOUR PRECEPTOR

As you begin your externship, strive to build a professional relationship with your preceptor. If the preceptor feels that you're a dedicated student, he will be more inclined to devote the time and energy into assisting you. Your preceptor was once where you are now, so he probably understands what you're going through. Make an effort to build a rapport with your preceptor, and he may be more willing to help you when you need it!

There are several things you can do to get to know your preceptor.

- Ask him how he prefers to be addressed. Some preceptors prefer a title (for example, "Mr. Jones"); others are comfortable with you using their first name.
- Ask how your preceptor got into the field of medical assisting, including where he went to school and what positions he has held. Remember, he may have professional contacts who can help you network and find a job later.
- Express interest in your tasks and ask the preceptor how he handles challenging situations. Ask, "How can I be a more successful medical assistant?"

DRESSING FOR SUCCESS

Looking your best promotes confidence and a positive attitude. Plus, feeling confident will encourage you to do a professional job. A messy, disheveled appearance gives the impression to others that you don't care about the work that you do.

For your externship, you may be asked to wear a uniform or follow a specific dress code. If the externship site requires clothing that differs from your school's requirements, you are usually asked to comply with the site's requirements. Here are some other helpful hints to consider when dressing for the externship.

- If you must wear a uniform, make sure it's freshly laundered and pressed. A clean but wrinkled uniform isn't acceptable.
- Avoid wearing clothing that is trendy or suggestive. This kind of clothing isn't appropriate for the externship site.
- Check your clothing to make sure it's in good condition, with no missing buttons, falling hems, rips, tears, or stains.
- Wear clean, appropriate shoes. Laced shoes look better with clean laces.
- If you wear nylon hosiery, check for runs and snags and replace as needed.
- If you have long hair, make sure it's pulled back from your face. Wash it often so that it looks and smells clean.
- If you wear makeup, keep it minimal and make sure it's tastefully applied.
- Avoid wearing perfume or cologne, as this can trigger an allergic reaction in some patients and coworkers.
- Keep fingernails short to avoid transferring pathogens (germs) or ripping gloves when you perform procedures.
- Wear only minimal, tasteful jewelry. Rings can puncture gloves, so it's a good idea to avoid wearing them to the externship site.
- Limit earrings to small studs, and check your facility's policy concerning the number of earrings that may be worn in each ear.
- Remove or conceal any body jewelry and cover any tattoos.

Your preceptor or clinical coordinator will inform you of the dress code in advance. Be sure to ask any questions you may have about dress before your externship begins.

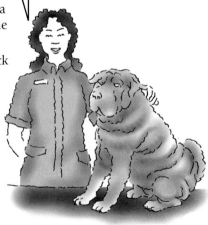

Wrinkles are cute on puppies, but not on uniforms. Be sure to iron those creases!

BEING THERE

Looking your best doesn't help you gain the experience you need unless you're regularly attending your externship sessions. It's important to plan on attending all your externship sessions so you can learn as much as you can and improve your skills. Also, the staff in the medical office depends on you, and it is important to be reliable. Remember that your attendance will be taken into account when the clinical coordinator makes her final evaluation.

Maintaining good health is essential because it will decrease your chance of catching an illness and having to call in sick. A healthy diet, regular exercise, and proper rest will give your immune system a boost. Careful attention to hygiene and medical asepsis, such as washing your hands before and after all procedures, will help you avoid bringing illnesses home from the externship site.

To maintain a good attendance record, you need to prepare to be ready and on time for every session. Here are some suggestions to help you do that.

- Office hours vary from site to site; it's always a good practice, however, to arrive a few minutes before the scheduled session. This allows time to check for phone messages, turn on office equipment, and gather any necessary materials.

- Plan your transportation ahead of time, and have a backup plan in case that fails.

- Leave plenty of time for any delays that might occur. Arriving at the site feeling frustrated by distractions, with no time to ease into the day, can cause anxiety and tension.

- Set aside time before each shift to mentally prepare. If you're feeling anxious or tense, it's more difficult to provide compassionate care to patients and deal with complex problems in the medical office.

ATTITUDE IS EVERYTHING

Your education has provided you with the knowledge and the technical skills you'll need to do your job. But no matter how good your technical skills are, having a poor attitude can make all the difference in your overall performance. During your externship, your attitude is reflected in:

- the way you perform each task
- your attendance
- your appearance

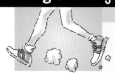

Running Smoothly

EXTERNSHIP PROTOCOL

What if you know you're going to be late or unable to attend a scheduled session?

If at any time you will be late or unable to attend a scheduled session, you must notify both the clinical coordinator and your preceptor. Almost all sites have an answering service for leaving messages. Memorize the site's phone number or program it into your cell phone. There is no excuse for failing to notify all parties involved if you will be late or absent.

> If for some reason you can't call in when you're going to be absent, have a friend or family member call in for you.

A positive attitude is infectious; when you project a positive attitude, others around you will begin to feel good also, and you will be better able to work together to accomplish your goals. On the flip side, a negative attitude has the exact opposite effect on patients and coworkers. When your attitude is negative, it makes others feel bad or unimportant. Make an extra effort to stay upbeat during your externship sessions. A positive attitude keeps you focused on what you're learning.

In part, your attitude is affected by how well you handle change and how adaptable and flexible you are when new or unusual situations arise. The medical profession is constantly changing, so you have to stay flexible to meet its demands. For example, in the classroom, you learned certain methods for treatments and procedures. But at the externship site, you may find yourself being asked to perform different procedures, either because the office uses newer technology, or simply because different offices perform the same tasks in slightly different ways. If you are not ready to adjust to change, you may begin to feel unsure of yourself or frustrated, and this could lead you to project a negative attitude.

Your attitude can determine how far you go in the medical field. Students who work with a positive attitude during their externship are more likely to reach higher levels of professional success than those who see the externship as a burden or difficulty.

Completing Tasks During Your Externship

Part of the medical externship is preparation, and the other part includes all the tasks you'll be asked to complete. But before you actually see a patient, you'll need to learn your way around the medical facility. Learning to adapt to the daily routines and procedures of the medical office will help make your externship a rewarding experience. Here are some things you'll learn:

- the medical office's layout
- coworkers' routines
- policies and procedures
- safety measures
- how to interact with coworkers
- how to interact with patients

LEARNING ABOUT THE OFFICE

It will be your responsibility to learn about the medical office in which you complete your externship. You can't always wait around for someone to tell you. Sometimes, you must decide to take action and get to know your environment. Make sure that you:

- become familiar with the office
- learn and follow office policies
- adhere to office safety procedures

Orientation

Each medical facility has its own way of doing things. The most efficient workers learn as much as they can about how their particular facility operates. So, it's important to orient yourself to the externship site where you'll be working. Doing so will help you provide better care and learn more as a student.

The following information is important to learn about your externship facility and may be included in a formal or informal orientation:

- the mission statement or goals of the medical facility
- fire and safety policies
- other emergency procedures
- standard precautions
- confidentiality rules
- computer access and password assignment (if applicable)

Here is a list of common questions you may wish to ask your preceptor or other office representative.

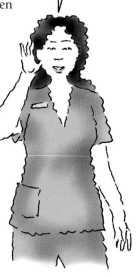

You'll be receiving a lot of information at first, so it's important to listen closely and take notes!

- Where may students park?
- Which building/door should I enter and exit through?
- Whom should I call if I'm going to be absent and when should the call be made?

Your preceptor or clinical coordinator will give you a schedule with the dates and times of your externship sessions. She will also explain written assignments and due dates. Be sure to ask questions if you don't understand something. Remember that the more information you gather, the more prepared you'll feel during your first externship session.

The Front Office

The first area of the medical office that you'll most likely encounter is the front office. You'll notice that the front of the facility is more like a typical office, with computers, phones, and fax machines. Get to know the front office staff; they will assist you as you learn your way around the office.

Here are some other tips to consider when learning your way around the front office.

- Learn how to use the equipment that may be unfamiliar to you, such as fax machines and copiers. If you need assistance, ask someone. Using this equipment improperly can break or damage it.
- Medical assistants complete a lot of paperwork. Learn the office's filing system, and learn how to handle patients' medical information. Know where to place folders and documents so they don't get lost and patient confidentiality is maintained.
- Seek out the resources you'll need to complete each task. Most medical offices have a room or closet where office supplies, such as pens and paper, are stored. Learn where it is, and ask about the procedure for accessing new materials.
- You may be asked to answer the phone. Know the procedures to use, such as answering with the proper greeting, placing a call on hold, and transferring a call to another staff member. Recognize emergency calls (you learned how to do this in Chapter 2) and handle them appropriately.

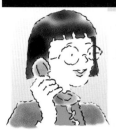

Ask The Professional ELECTRONIC DEVICES

Q: *I like to use my MP3 player when I'm working. Listening to music helps me relax. Can I use these devices during my externship?*

A: Using your MP3 player while you work or study at home is fine, but using these devices in a professional medical office is unacceptable. Just as you wouldn't take a cell phone call while talking with a patient, you shouldn't use electronic devices that can be distracting to others. And when you're wearing your headphones, patients and coworkers may feel uncomfortable approaching you. If you're having trouble concentrating during your externship, then try some of the relaxation techniques previously discussed in this chapter.

Office Policies

You'll also learn about the facility's *policies.* Policies are sets of general principles that must be followed. Maintaining patient confidentiality is an example of a policy; it's a goal that the facility strives for. The facility's *procedures* are based on these policies. Procedures describe a specific way in which each task should be performed. Returning all patient documents to a locked file cabinet is an example of a procedure that results from the policy of protecting confidentiality.

Your externship facility should have a policies and procedures manual. Know where this manual is located and refer to it often. Even though you learned a procedure one way in the classroom, the facility may have another method. Understanding and following your externship site's policies and procedures will make you a thoughtful and effective medical assistant in training.

Safety Procedures

The medical facility's policies and procedures are often created with the intention of keeping you and other staff and patients safe. Patients' safety is the responsibility of all members of the health care team—don't forget that this team now includes you! Be sure to familiarize yourself with the office's policies and procedures concerning safety. If you don't understand something, ask someone! It's better to be safe than sorry.

Keeping Germs at Bay

The risk of infection is always present when you work with patients. The Centers for Disease Control and Prevention (CDC) has created a set of guidelines to provide the widest possible protection against the transmission of infection. Follow these guidelines to protect yourself and patients.

- Wash your hands before and after patient care, after removing gloves, and immediately after you have contact with a patient's blood or body fluid.

- Wear gloves if you will or could come into contact with blood or other body fluids, specimens, mucous membranes, broken skin, or contaminated objects or surfaces.

- Change gloves and wash your hands between seeing patients. When caring for the same patient, change gloves and wash your hands if you touch anything with a high concentration of microorganisms.

- Wear a fluid-resistant gown, eye protection, and a mask during procedures that are likely to generate droplets of blood or body fluid.

- Carefully handle used patient care equipment that's soiled with blood or body fluids. Follow facility guidelines for cleaning and disinfecting equipment and surfaces.

- Handle needles and sharps carefully and immediately discard in the appropriate containers after use.

- Immediately notify your supervisor if you are injured by a needle or other sharp instrument, or if you have broken skin that becomes contaminated with a patient's blood or other body fluid. Your supervisor will begin the appropriate investigation and provide necessary medical care for the incident.

- If occupational exposure to blood is likely, get the hepatitis B vaccine series.

Avoiding Equipment Injuries

Injuries due to negligent use of equipment are preventable. You're responsible for making sure the equipment you use for patient care is free from defects. Before performing or assisting with a procedure, make sure all the necessary equipment is present (not lost or missing) and in good condition (no damages or breaks). Report any possible defects to your supervisor immediately. You're also responsible for using all equipment properly, according to the externship site's policy and procedures manual. If you're unsure of a procedure, ask your preceptor for guidance.

Avoiding Other Injuries

Other injuries that can occur in the medical office include:

- back injuries
- chemical injuries
- injuries from a fall

Back injuries are common because many patient care activities require you to push, pull, lift, and carry. Use proper body mechanics to reduce the risk of injuring yourself and patients.

- Flex your hips and knees instead of bending at the waist. This position distributes weight evenly and helps maintain balance.
- Spread your feet apart.
- Move your feet, rather than twisting and bending at the waist.

Chemical injuries can happen in the medical office because of the routine use of potentially hazardous chemicals. Powerful cleaning solutions and disinfectants are the common culprits. A Material Safety Data Sheet (MSDS) provides you with information about the physical and chemical hazards that can occur from these substances. Each MSDS provides information about chemicals and how to treat exposure to the substances. Know where these forms are stored in the facility where you'll be working.

It's important to take measures to protect yourself and patients from falling. Some patients have an increased risk for falls, especially if they're elderly or if they're taking certain medications. Here are some tips to avoid falls.

- Make sure there are no pieces of furniture or other objects obstructing hallways or walkways in the waiting room.
- Provide adequate lighting and a clean, clutter-free area.
- Be aware of all patients who are taking medications that could increase their risk of falling.
- Assist the patient when walking, especially if he's using a cane or has other mobility issues.
- Quickly and effectively clean spills that can make the floor slippery.

Remember that safety is everyone's business, so take it seriously and be informed. It's better to ask someone about the proper safety procedures than to risk infection or injury. And if you make a mistake, tell someone immediately! Protect yourself and patients at all times.

> Spread your feet apart and bend at the knees to prevent back injuries

INTERACTING WITH COWORKERS

During the clinical orientation, your preceptor or clinical coordinator will introduce you to staff members. This is the perfect opportunity to make a good impression. It's also an opportunity to learn the various roles of each member of the health care team, as well as to learn to work with many different personalities.

You'll begin to learn that each team member has a unique set of skills and abilities, and each individual has a vital role to play within the office. Remember to show an enthusiastic attitude when you interact with coworkers. Take a humble approach, realizing that you have much to learn from every member of the staff. Show respect to each member of the team and appreciate the jobs they do.

What's the Routine?

As a medical assistant in training with little experience, it will be your responsibility to learn how the office runs on a daily basis. For example, who opens up the waiting room and greets patients? Is the office closed for lunch, or does the staff alternate breaks? Who cleans examination rooms between patients? It's important to follow all physicians' and other health care professionals' instructions. They have the experience and know-how to get the job done well, so follow their lead. If you're unsure of something, ask for clarification.

Remember the three "Ls" when adapting to the medical facility's daily routine.

- *Look.* Watch other staff members as they go about their daily routines, and observe how each job is related to the others to understand how the staff works as a team.

- *Listen.* Keep an ear out for key terms or phrases repeated throughout the day. Pay attention when a staff member explains something or gives directions.

- *Learn.* Incorporate your observations by practicing skills and techniques. If you make a mistake, try again or ask someone to help you.

There Is No "I" in Team

As you learn the ropes of the medical office, you'll also learn how the staff works as a team. Team members have a common goal, and they work together to achieve it. Every team member steps up and contributes his own skills and talents to get the job done.

A team is only as good as its weakest member. That means everyone has to give 100 percent so the medical team can perform at its very best level. Show interest in being a part of the team. Learn how to pitch in and help without being asked, and work cooperatively with others to get the job done. Offer ideas, but don't expect to be the leader of every task. Remember that you're there to learn from experienced others, so you should listen and observe instead of trying to run the show!

Remember that a team is made up of equal individuals. Every individual is important and should be heard and recognized. Some tasks are solitary and require concentration and quiet. But your performance on most of the tasks you complete in the office will depend on your ability and willingness to work with others. You'll enjoy the externship a lot more and you'll get more out of it if you become a team player.

> Part of teamwork involves knowing your limitations. Sometimes, you should watch and learn from the sidelines

Accountability

Although you'll be part of a team of health care professionals during your externship, you'll still be accountable for your own actions. You'll also be accountable for your own learning. How much you get out of your externship depends on your willingness to learn and ask questions.

The following guidelines will help you maintain accountability during the externship.

- Show up at your externship site on time, with a professional appearance and a positive attitude. Be ready for whatever comes your way.

- If you're going to be absent, demonstrate accountability by calling the designated phone number at the appropriate time and making up any missed work within the given time frame.

- Never try to perform a skill you're unsure about or use a piece of equipment you haven't been taught to operate.

- Admit to your mistakes. Never blame something you did on someone else. Coworkers will appreciate your honesty. Learn from your mistakes, and then move on.

- Ask for help. The medical staff will be glad to answer any questions you have and offer advice. Most people will remember what it was like to be a student and will be glad to help you!

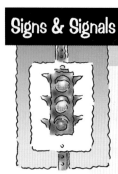

Signs & Signals

MAKING THE MOST OF YOUR EXTERNSHIP EXPERIENCE

How much you get out of your externship experience depends on how much you put into it. Your skills and enthusiasm for learning will keep your externship going smoothly. Here are some ways to make sure that you get the most out of your externship experience.

- Show enthusiasm and interest in learning.
- Be curious and ask lots of questions.
- Work well and cooperate with others.
- Offer to assist with as many tasks as possible.
- Ask for clarification before performing any procedure that you're unsure of.
- Immediately admit to any errors or mistakes you make.
- Accept constructive criticism from staff members.
- Show initiative. Anticipate tasks that need to be done, and do them before you're asked.
- Avoid making negative or pessimistic remarks, such as "I will never learn to do this," or, "This office is outdated."

- Communicate all concerns to a staff member. If you or someone else breaks a policy or procedure, be accountable by letting someone else know.

When your coworkers feel that you're accountable and trustworthy, they will trust you with larger matters, such as more complex procedures or tasks. In this way, you'll learn more and get more out of the externship experience.

CARING FOR PATIENTS

You finally have the opportunity to work with actual patients, and you may be feeling a little nervous. It's okay to feel this way at first. But be encouraged! You've practiced your skills, and now you're ready to use them in an actual medical office. Learning to care for patients includes knowing how to use equipment properly and being able to maintain patient confidentiality by following HIPAA rules.

Know the Equipment

The back office is the part of the facility that includes a lot of medical equipment. This is where most procedures and treatments take place.

The equipment you'll use, such as ECG machines for performing electrocardiograms and autoclaves for sterilizing equipment, may be operated slightly differently than the way you learned in the classroom. Be willing and flexible to learn new procedures for operating this equipment. Saying, "My school didn't teach me this," communicates to others that you're unable or unwilling to adapt your skills according to the facility's needs. When using medical equipment, it's also important that you follow the appropriate office procedures to protect the safety of yourself and patients. Consult the office's policy and procedures manual if you're unsure of how to operate a piece of equipment.

Maintain Patient Confidentiality

Caring for patients also includes maintaining patient confidentiality. As you learned previously in Chapter 1, HIPAA is the Health Insurance Portability and Accountability Act. It's a federal law that protects the privacy, confidentiality, and security of all medical information. During your externship, you'll receive information about maintaining patient rights under HIPAA that's specifically tailored to the health care facility where you'll be working. Failure to comply with HIPAA, whether it's intentional or not, could result in legal action being taken against the medical office.

HIPAA is like the medical constitution—it requires that you uphold and defend patients' privacy rights.

The following are some practices you should incorporate to uphold patient privacy.

- Protect your computer password. Avoid sharing your password with anyone.
- Log off the computer when you're finished.
- Keep patients' charts closed when not in use.
- Avoid leaving faxes and computer printouts unattended.
- Don't discuss patient information for any reason other than learning. Don't discuss patient information with family and friends. Don't gossip about a patient with other staff members.
- Keep your voice down when talking with the physician about a patient. Don't discuss a patient's information with other patients or visitors without the patient's consent.

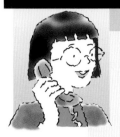

Ask The Professional

RECOGNIZING AND RESPONDING TO CONFIDENTIALITY ISSUES

Q: *My coworkers routinely discuss confidential patient information during lunch breaks. They've asked me questions about patients whom I've cared for. I'm new to the office, but their behavior seems unacceptable to me. What should I do?*

A: You're absolutely right; discussing patient information, unless it is for a medical reason, is unethical. Your coworkers are jeopardizing the privacy of their patients. Don't join in as they're gossiping, and don't answer their questions. I would suggest discussing this matter in private with your preceptor or other supervisor. They'll take the necessary actions to stop this behavior.

- Remove any *patient identifiers* (such as a patient's name, Social Security number, or address) before handing in written class work.

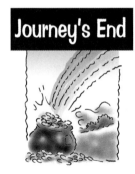

Journey's End

- The purpose of the externship experience is to practice and refine the skills that you'll use as a medical assistant.
- The different types of externship facilities include family or general practices and specialty practices.
- The externship is a valuable experience because it gives you the opportunity to work with and learn from professionals in the field.
- You can prepare mentally for the externship by learning ways to avoid anxiety and reduce stress.
- Physical preparation for the externship includes maintaining a healthy, balanced diet; exercising regularly; getting enough rest; and being sure to get the required vaccinations.
- To prepare professionally for the externship, use time management strategies, establish priorities, and enlist the help of your family members and friends.
- Make a good impression during your externship by having a positive attitude, a professional appearance, and an excellent attendance record.

- Use the same good habits that worked for you in the classroom so your externship will be just as successful.

- The key tasks and expectations involved in the externship program include learning how to work in the medical office, how to interact with coworkers, and how to care for patients.

- Protect patients' privacy rights by adhering to HIPAA policies and procedures.

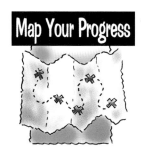
Map Your Progress

Answer the following multiple-choice questions.

1. What does a *preceptor* do?
   a. instructs your class
   b. acts as your mentor
   c. grades your performance
   d. provides your financial support

2. An example of a specialty practice is:
   a. a general practice.
   b. a dermatology practice.
   c. a family practice.
   d. all of the above

3. As a student, how can you benefit from your externship experience?
   a. You will have a chance to earn some extra money.
   b. You will have the opportunity to teach coworkers the latest skills and techniques you've learned in the classroom.
   c. You will gain valuable hands-on experience working in a medical facility.
   d. none of the above

4. How can you prepare mentally for the externship?
   a. Enlist the help of your family and friends.
   b. Get in the habit of going to bed and waking up at the same time every day.
   c. Eat a healthy breakfast every morning.
   d. Find ways to avoid anxiety and reduce your stress level.

5. What can you do during your externship to make it a positive experience?
   a. Be a curious learner and ask lots of questions.
   b. Observe other staff members as they carry out their daily tasks and offer constructive criticism.
   c. Point out equipment in the office that looks outdated.
   d. Immediately correct any errors or mistakes you make without drawing attention to them.

6. Why should you keep your fingernails short during the externship?
   a. to avoid angry stares from patients
   b. to avoid dropping sterile equipment
   c. to avoid transferring pathogens or ripping gloves
   d. to avoid chipping a nail

7. *Policies* are:
   a. sets of general principles that must be followed.
   b. guidelines to help you control patients.
   c. step-by-step instructions for certain tasks.
   d. lists of rules to help you protect patients' privacy.

8. During your externship, how can you protect your own safety as well as the safety of patients?
   a. by washing your hands frequently to prevent the spread of infection
   b. by knowing where the MSDS forms are stored in case of accidental exposure to a chemical substance
   c. by using proper body mechanics when lifting or moving heavy objects
   d. all of the above

9. Admitting to your mistakes shows that you are:
   a. accountable.
   b. skilled.
   c. empathetic.
   d. organized.

10. How can you uphold patients' privacy as you go about your tasks in the medical office?
    a. Only discuss private medical information with a patient's immediate family members and close friends.
    b. Keep your voice down when talking with the physician about a patient.
    c. Be sure to add patient identifiers to any written class work you're asked to submit.
    d. Share your computer password with other office staff members, but avoid letting patients overhear it.

Chapter 6

LANDING YOUR MEDICAL ASSISTING JOB

Road Map to Success

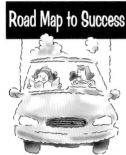

- Identify possible obstacles to employment as a medical assistant, and explain how to overcome them

- Explain how to determine your ideal medical assisting job

- Establish realistic goals for your future

- Describe basic job search methods, including how best to utilize available resources

- Create effective resumes and cover letters, and explain the benefits of these job search tools

- Explain how effective communication skills and proper interviewing techniques will assist you in getting hired as a medical assistant

- List the factors to consider when deciding whether to accept or decline a job offer

Chapter Competencies

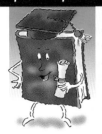

- Use correct grammar, spelling, and formatting techniques in written works (ABHES 2.j.)

- Demonstrate fundamental writing skills (ABHES 2.o.)

- Respond to and initiate written communications (CAAHEP 3.c.1.a.)

- Project a positive attitude (ABHES 1.a.)

You've worked hard as a student and during your externship, and now it's time to enter the workforce as a medical assistant. Armed with the right information, you can be optimistic and self-assured when conducting your job search. This positive attitude will help you overcome obstacles along your journey. In this chapter, you'll learn how to do the following:

- determine which job is right for you
- search and apply for positions
- prepare for job interviews to ensure that they go smoothly
- decide whether to accept or decline employers' offers

Overcoming Obstacles

Maybe you're reentering the workforce or perhaps you're seeking your first job. Regardless of your employment background, one thing is for certain: you have now acquired the skills and training necessary to land a great job in the medical field!

BEING A FIRST-TIME WORKER

If this is your first time looking for a job, congratulations! You've gained valuable knowledge and experience during your schooling and externship, and now you're ready to find a medical assisting position.

You may be nervous about the job search itself and wondering how to go about finding the job that you want. The good news is that there are many available resources designed to help you find the right job. You'll learn about these resources later in this chapter.

If you're worried about your lack of work experience, try thinking about this particular obstacle in a positive light. Your inexperience can be an asset, too. For example, at this point in your career, you've dealt with few or no setbacks or problems on the job, so you may have more energy and willingness to meet these challenges head-on. You're also coming to the position with few biases, so you're open to new

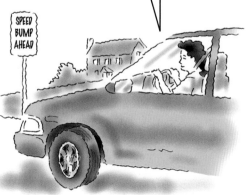

It's helpful to ask for advice from friends and family members who've searched for jobs. They may be able to offer suggestions and help you avoid "bumps in the road."

ideas and different ways of working. Some employers seek out new graduates so they can train them in a specific way. Your optimistic, fresh approach to the profession of medical assisting will make employers sit up and take notice.

REENTERING THE WORKFORCE

Reentering the workforce involves a different set of obstacles, such as:

- explaining gaps in your employment to prospective employers
- seeking a new position after being fired or laid off from a previous job
- transitioning from one career to another

You may have been out of work for six months or six years, depending on your particular circumstances. Regardless of the length of your absence, reentering the workforce can be a stressful, yet exciting, time in your life.

Before you begin your job search, consider the ways in which a new job will affect your daily schedule and existing priorities. You may need to sit down with your family and explain how these changes might affect them. Recruiting the support of your family and friends will help you prepare for the necessary adjustments to your schedule. And the help and encouragement of people who care about you will ensure a smooth transition as you reenter the workforce.

"Minding the Gaps" in Your Employment

You may have gaps in your employment due to:

- schooling
- relocation
- pregnancy
- illness
- other changes in life circumstances

Potential employers want to see that you're a dedicated and consistent worker, and they may ask you to explain any lapses in employment. Try to put a positive spin on any unfortunate occurrences. For example, if you left a job because you couldn't balance your professional and private life, you might say something like, "I left because I wanted to take some time to refocus my goals and determine the type of work atmosphere where I would be happiest and most successful." This shows that you took a proactive role in directing your career. This type of honest self-awareness will be respected and admired by a potential employer.

However, being honest doesn't mean you have to share personal details that you may be uncomfortable discussing. Employees sometimes leave their previous jobs for reasons that may be negative, embarrassing, or private, such as mental illness or family tragedy. In these or similar circumstances, it might be best to simply explain that you left your previous position for personal reasons. Show your enthusiasm for the new direction your career is taking, and reassure potential employers that you're ready for a new challenge.

Being Laid Off

You may be reentering the workforce after being laid off. Downsizing is a common cause for layoffs, and unsatisfactory job performance isn't a factor in these situations. Explain to potential employers the reasons why you were laid off and emphasize your positive behavior. If you stayed with a company despite the risk of being laid off, it shows that you're a loyal employee who cares about the work you do. Both are positive qualities that potential employers often seek.

Being Fired

Everyone makes mistakes at one point or another. Mistakes are a part of life, and they help us grow as individuals. Unfortunately, your work history might contain mistakes that are potentially damaging to your record, such as being fired from a previous job. But a past firing is no reason to quit searching for a new job. In fact, these potential weak spots on your resume can be strengths if you've learned from your experience.

You can't run from your mistakes, but you *can* learn from them!

If a potential employer asks why you were fired, be honest. Lying or embellishing will only cause problems for you down the road. Avoid blaming your supervisors or coworkers for the firing. Own up to your mistakes, and explain to your potential employer what the experience taught you and how you will improve your job performance if you're hired.

Making a Career Change

Transitioning from one career to another shows that you have the courage to take risks and follow your dreams. Maybe you were unhappy with your previous career, or maybe you're just looking for a new challenge. Whatever the case, switching careers can be a very intense time. You've completed the necessary schooling and training, and you're ready to begin working as a medical assistant. But perhaps you're wondering if employers will want to hire you. After all, you might not have any direct experience in the medical field. What skills will you bring to your new job?

The fact is that you may be bringing many skills from your previous positions that are relevant to medical assisting. For example, if you worked as an administrative assistant, you'll be using some of the same technical and customer service skills as a medical assistant. Your former job experiences make you a diverse employee who can bring a fresh approach to the job. Keep that in mind as you begin your job search.

Setting Goals

After you've completed your externship, you might have a better understanding of what you want out of a job. For example, you may know that you'd like working at an obstetrics office because you enjoyed working in this specialty field during your externship. Decide what you need and want from a job, and make that your goal. Working toward a goal will make the job search a lot easier to handle because you'll have focused and narrowed your options. You can also determine the right job for you by doing the following:

- analyzing your strengths and weaknesses
- paying attention to your ideals
- setting career goals

SELF-ANALYSIS

To get the job that you want, you have to first know who you are. Job hunting starts with self-analysis. What kinds of things are you good at? The job interview is your chance to sell yourself to a potential employer, so you have to know what makes you special. These are your strengths, the aspects of your character and job performance that will make you a valuable employee. When you're interviewing for a position, concentrate on communicating your strengths to the interviewer.

You should also understand your weaknesses. Weaknesses are the things that you're actively working to improve or refine. Weaknesses can often be used as something positive. For example, you may find that you procrastinate and wait to do things until the last minute because you work better under pressure. Although procrastination is a weakness, the ability to work well under pressure will come in handy should you face any emergency situations in the medical office.

Take an honest look at your strengths and weaknesses and make a list to better understand who you are as an employee. Your instructors, preceptor, friends, and family members may also be able to shed light on your strengths and weaknesses. Talk openly and honestly with these individuals and listen to what they have to say. Sometimes, it's difficult to realize in which areas or tasks you excel or fall short. Other people's perspectives can help you see yourself in a new light. Once you understand your strengths and weaknesses, it's time to start looking for the right job.

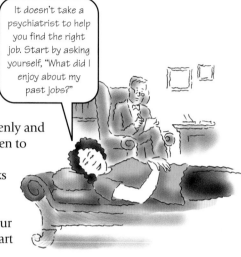

It doesn't take a psychiatrist to help you find the right job. Start by asking yourself, "What did I enjoy about my past jobs?"

DETERMINING YOUR IDEAL JOB

You can't wait around and hope that the right job will just land in your lap; you have to make it happen. In fact, you'll work harder and be happier if you choose your own workplace.

When determining your ideal job, consider the following aspects:

- specialty area (e.g., obstetrics, pediatrics, surgery)
- duties (clinical or administrative)
- type of employer and supervisor
- other employees and coworkers
- type of facility
- desired atmosphere (casual or formal)
- ideal hours
- availability of flextime (scheduling that allows for a personal choice in hours or days worked)

Although you want to be happy with your job, remember that sometimes you'll have to compromise a little. For example, the job itself may be great, but your daily commute would be long, or the starting salary might be low, but you'd have opportunities for advancement.

CAREER GOALS

Setting career goals helps you be proactive. You can find the job you really want, instead of settling for the first position you come across. Think about the type of job you want and the career direction you'd like to follow *before* you begin searching advertisements for available positions. If you start with a set goal, you're more likely to find what you're looking for.

In terms of position and income, where would you like to be in two years? In five years? Set goals related to the type of facility where you want to work, which tasks you'd like to perform, and the career direction you want to take. You can find information about medical assisting and other professions on the Department of Labor's website: www.dol.gov. Search the *Occupational Outlook Handbook* by typing a job title, such as "medical assistant," in the search bar. The site provides information about the required training, average salary, working conditions, and job prospects for each occupation listed in its database. Here is some information about the profession of medical assisting that might be of interest to you.

- Because the health care industry is growing (due to advances in technology and the aging population), the profession of medical assisting is growing, too. In fact, the Department of Labor estimates that medical assisting will be one of the fastest growing occupations over the next several years.

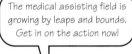

The medical assisting field is growing by leaps and bounds. Get in on the action now!

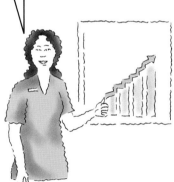

- More than half of all medical assisting jobs are in physicians' offices. A variety of other types of facilities also employ medical assistants, including specialty facilities, government agencies, laboratories, and schools.

- Like many other occupations, factors such as skill level, formal training, experience, and geographic location affect the salaries of medical assistants.

Job Search Methods and Resources

Searching for a job today can be as easy as clicking on a mouse. There are many resources and methods of searching for a job, so you can choose which ones work best for you. Here are a few of the options available to you:

- networking
- visiting your school placement office
- looking in industry publications

- answering online and newspaper advertisements
- consulting private, temporary, or government agencies

Exploring some of the methods and resources available to you will help you get your foot in the door!

NETWORKING

You've probably heard the phrase, "In show business, it's all about who you know." You may not be auditioning for a Broadway musical, but having good contacts is useful when you're looking for a job in any field.

During your time as a student, you'll meet people and build as many contacts within the medical field as possible. Your externship probably helped you learn how to network. **Networking** is using friends, family members, and professional colleagues to advance or obtain information in the workplace. You can never have too many contacts. Make a list of the people you know who have the right contacts for your job search and let them know that you're seeking employment. Friends and acquaintances might be able to help you secure an interview with a potential employer. Just remember that your contacts can provide you with information about a job only if they know you're searching.

> Professional associations can sometimes give you the "inside scoop" on finding a job in the health care field.

SCHOOL PLACEMENT OFFICE

Find out if your school has a career placement office. This office can be an invaluable resource when you're trying to find a job. If your school has a placement office, contact the coordinator or personnel officer and explain what you're looking for and where you want to work. These staff members can assist you with securing an interview or position. To obtain better results, try to establish a good working relationship with your contact at the placement office. Be sure to arrive for scheduled meetings on time and stay in touch with your contact at the office during the length of your job search.

PROFESSIONAL ASSOCIATIONS

Professional associations, such as the American Association of Medical Assistants (AAMA), can sometimes provide you with information about job opportunities in your area. Visit the AAMA's official website at www.aama-ntl.org to locate your state and local chapter. Your local chapter will be able to refer you to an appropriate contact person.

NEWSPAPERS

When searching for a job, the first place many people turn to is the newspaper. This is a good idea; newspapers are easy to find and filled with job listings. When responding to a newspaper advertisement, follow these guidelines.

- Be sure to do exactly what the advertisement asks you to do. One of the qualities that many interviewers look for is the ability to follow directions.
- Try to make your response stand out from the others, yet remain professional. (See *Writing Effective Cover Letters.*)
- Remember that the medical profession projects an image of care and friendliness. Seek to project this image in your response.

THE INTERNET

You may also find job listings on the Internet. Many large medical practices list job opportunities on their websites. You can respond to these advertisements by e-mailing or calling the provider directly. You'll most likely be asked to direct your response to the office manager or human resources department. Be careful to follow directions when responding to these postings. Similar to newspaper advertisements, online postings usually indicate how you should respond to or apply for the position.

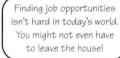

Finding job opportunities isn't hard in today's world. You might not even have to leave the house!

Other facilities advertise available positions on popular job search sites. (See page 190 for a listing of popular and federal job search sites.)

The American Medical Technologists (AMT) maintains its own job search site, the AMT Career Connection. This site can be accessed from the AMT's home page: www.amt1.com. The AMT Career Connection allows candidates to post their resumes online and search for available jobs within their field. When answering online advertisements, adhere to the same guidelines that you would follow when responding to newspaper advertisements. Following directions, accentuating your skills and accomplishments, and projecting a professional image will help your response stand out from the rest.

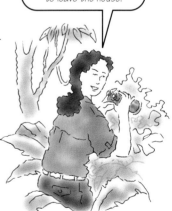

PRIVATE AGENCIES

Many medical facilities hire private agencies to interview and screen potential candidates. This helps busy medical offices avoid

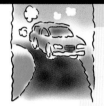

Road Rules

POPULAR AND FEDERAL JOB SEARCH SITES

The following websites can provide you with some help when searching for the right job:

- www.ajb.org
- www.CareerBuilder.com
- www.certmedassistant.com
- www.flipdog.com
- hotjobs.yahoo.com
- www.indeed.com
- www.jobbankusa.com
- www.jobcentral.com
- www.jobster.com
- www.monster.com
- www.simplyhired.com
- www.usajobs.opm.gov

receiving too many applications from unqualified applicants. A fee is charged for the service but is usually paid by the employer.

Your school's career placement office should have contact information for the placement agencies in your area. Call the agency to make an appointment with a representative who will interview you and explain the procedure for applying.

STATE AND LOCAL EMPLOYMENT OFFICES

Government-run employment offices are designed to find work for the unemployed. You can search the Web to find your state's office. These offices frequently have job listings that you won't find anywhere else. Instead of calling the office, make an appointment to visit and register with the service. Get to know a contact person who will help you look for the right job.

TEMPORARY AGENCIES

Temporary agencies, or "temp" agencies, fill short-term vacancies for medical offices. If you are new to an area, finding a position through a temp agency is a good way to learn which facilities might be a good fit for you. You may be assigned to a

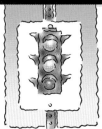

Signs & Signals — POSTING YOUR RESUME ON THE WEB

Most job search sites allow you to conduct a search for jobs in your area. You can do so by simply entering the title of the position you're seeking and any other relevant keywords into the search bar. But did you know that some sites not only allow job seekers to search advertisements; they also allow potential employers to search for qualified candidates? Right now, your next employer might be searching for a candidate like *you!*

Popular job search sites, such as CareerBuilder.com, give job seekers the option to post their resumes online. It's usually a very simple process.

1. First, click on the appropriate "Post Resume" link.

2. Next, click on "Browse" to locate your resume file on the computer. If you're using a computer in your campus library or computer laboratory, insert the disk or CD containing your resume file before clicking on "Browse."

3. Finally, upload your file to the website by clicking on "Upload."

Your resume will then be added to the site's searchable resume database. Potential employers may access this database to search for candidates who meet their qualifications.

certain office or health care facility for several days or several weeks. If you enjoy the work and like the facility, leave your resume with the appropriate individuals and let them know that you're interested in working there full-time if a position becomes available. Check with the temp agency regarding any fees that you may be charged or that the medical office may have to pay if it hires you (often called a finder's fee).

The Application Process

Once you've found a position that you're interested in, the next step is to apply. The application process usually includes these steps:

- submitting your resume
- submitting a cover letter
- completing an employment application

During this process, keep a journal of your job search activity. Doing so will help you remember where you've applied, what positions you've applied for, and when you submitted your resume, cover letter, and employment application. This record will provide you with an idea of the direction your job search is taking. It will also keep you organized. After all, you don't want to apply for the same job twice!

CREATING YOUR RESUME

Writing your resume can seem like a daunting task. Where do you begin? What should you include? There are many resources available to help you answer these questions.

Start with your school library. Most schools have books on how to create resumes. If you'd like to take a more direct approach, you can consult your school's career office. A career counselor will be able to help you organize and write down your information in the proper format. You can also consult websites, which are usually filled with free information. However, some sites charge fees. Focus on obtaining free resources before paying for these services. Many word processing programs have templates for resumes. Save your resume on a disk or CD, and be sure to customize it for the position you're seeking. Keep tweaking the information so that it is personalized for each interview.

All About You

Your resume is a portrait of you. It should accurately reflect who you are as a student, your career goals and experience, and your skills and abilities. Include the following information in your resume.

- *Contact information.* Include your name, address, phone number, and professional e-mail address at the top of your resume. These items are usually centered at the top of the page.
- *Education.* Start by listing the most recent school you've attended (and any degree, diploma, or certificate you earned there) and work backward in time. Include major areas of study.
- *Affiliations or volunteer work.* If this information shows you have organizational and leadership skills, you should include it.
- *Experience.* List your work experience, such as an externship or previous position(s) held. Be sure to detail the skills you acquired and any relevant responsibilities or tasks you carried out.
- *References.* Your references will usually be included on a separate sheet. On your resume, write "References available

upon request." (References are discussed in greater detail later in this chapter.)

- *Credentials.* Your CMA or RMA credentials are important to include in your resume. In today's competitive job market, your credentials set you apart from the crowd.

When detailing your experience, you may choose one of two standard formats: functional or chronological. A *functional* resume focuses on your skills and qualifications rather than your employment history. This format works well for recent graduates, those who are making a career change, those who have employment gaps, or those who are reentering the workforce after a significant absence. A *chronological* resume is useful if you have an employment history, particularly if the history is relevant to the position you're currently seeking. To format your experience chronologically, start with your most recent employment and work backward. Include your dates of employment, title, and a few of your key responsibilities for each position you've held.

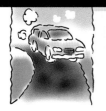

Road Rules   AND . . . ACTION!

As you create your resume, it's important to highlight your accomplishments and to make your skills and experience stand out. You can do this by using action words, such as the following:

- achieved
- assisted
- attained
- completed
- composed
- conducted
- created
- developed
- directed
- ensured
- established
- filed
- generated
- handled

- implemented
- maintained
- operated
- organized
- participated
- performed
- planned
- prepared
- processed
- scheduled
- screened
- selected
- solved
- wrote

Tina Elmwood, C.M.A.
22 Brandy Drive
Dayton, Ohio 12345
937-555-0101

Employment Objective: To use my medical assisting skills in a challenging position. My goal is to work with children. (*Change this sentence to reflect the type of office that you are applying to.*)

Experience:

Externship (160 hours) at Family Practice Associates, Bayview Drive, Dayton, Ohio (*If you have a positive evaluation from your preceptor, bring it with you to the interview. Do not attach it to the resume.*)

Education:

Medical Assisting Program, Diploma. Graduated June 2008. West County Community College, Dayton, Ohio (*Bring a copy of your diploma and transcripts to the interview. Do not attach them unless employer has specifically requested them.*)
Dayton High School, Diploma. Graduated June 2006. Dayton, Ohio

Skills:

Clinical and Laboratory skills listed on Role Delineation for Medical Assisting

Administrative skills listed on Role Delineation for Medical Assisting

Comfortable using all types of standard office equipment

Familiar with XYZ software programs (*List software programs that you are comfortable with. If you know what type of software the office uses, list that as well.*)

Certifications:

Certified Medical Assistant, American Association of Medical Assistants (*Bring copy to interview or attach to resume.*)
Cardiopulmonary Resuscitation, American Heart Association (*Bring copy to interview or attach to resume.*)

References available upon request.

A functional resume focuses on your skills and qualifications rather than employment history. This format works well for recent graduates and applicants who are reentering the workforce after a number of years.

Beatrice Meza, C.M.A.
123 Main Street
West Hartford, Connecticut 54321
860-555-0199

Employment Objective: To use my medical assisting skills in a challenging position. My goal is to work in an obstetrical office. (*Change this sentence to reflect the type of office that you are applying to.*)

Education:

2007–2008 Medical Assisting Program; Mountain Laurel Community College, West Hartford, Connecticut (*Bring a copy of your diploma and transcripts to the interview. Do not attach them unless employer has specifically requested them.*)

Externship:

July 2008–(160 hours) Women's Health Care Center, Hartford, Connecticut (*If you have a positive evaluation from your preceptor, bring it with you to the interview. Do not attach it to the resume.*)

Work Experience:

July 2007–present Receptionist, Dermatology Consultants, West Hartford, Connecticut. Worked part time while I was in school. Answered and triaged telephone calls. Assisted with various other medical administrative responsibilities. (*If you have a reference letter from this employer, bring it with you to the interview. Be prepared to answer questions about why you are leaving this position.*)
May 2004–July 2007 Cashier/Clerk for SuperMarket Grocers, West Hartford, Connecticut. Worked part time. Responsible for training new employees. Promoted to senior cashier.

Skills:

Clinical and Laboratory skills listed on the Role Delineation for Medical Assisting

Administrative skills listed on the Role Delineation for Medical Assisting

Comfortable using all types of standard office equipment

Familiar with XYZ software programs (*List software programs that you are comfortable with. If you know what type of software the office uses, list that as well.*)

Activities/Honors

Student Government representative

Most Improved Medical Assisting Student in 2007

References available upon request.

A chronological resume is useful if you have an employment history, particularly if the history is relevant to the position you're currently seeking. It is useful to those who have a lengthy work history.

Style and Substance

Your resume is like a speech; it's not just about what you say, but how you say it. Here are some tips to help you create a professional resume.

- Limit your resume to one page. Include only the information the reviewer needs to know.
- Avoid including hobbies and personal interests unless they're related to the position you're seeking. It is not relevant that you play in a band, but it would be impressive to know that you volunteer at a free clinic.
- Use action words. Action words are strong verbs, such as "achieved," "organized," and "participated." (See *And . . . Action!*)
- Be honest. Don't embellish or fictionalize your resume. This is unethical and will lead to problems later.

Your resume should look professional and neat. Once you're ready to type the resume, follow these steps.

1. Keep a one-inch margin around the text. Single space within the sections of information but leave a blank line between each section.
2. Be sure to use regular type. Avoid fonts that are cute or decorative. Print your resume in black ink.
3. Ask someone to proofread your work. It can be difficult to find your own errors and another pair of eyes may catch something that you miss.
4. Print the resume on 8.5-by-11-inch white or off-white heavy bond paper. Avoid using colored or thin paper as this won't create a professional appearance.
5. Mail the resume in an 8.5-by-11-inch manila envelope. This will present the interviewer with a resume and cover letter that are neat and smooth, with no fold lines.

WRITING EFFECTIVE COVER LETTERS

When contacting a prospective employer, you'll need to send a cover letter along with your resume. The cover letter is like your calling card; it gives the reader a small sample of yourself and what you have to offer. The cover letter should be brief but meaningful. You want the letter to impress the reader, so choose your words wisely. Here are some other tips to consider when constructing your cover letter.

- Be sure to mention the job itself in your letter. You may consider making a forthright statement, such as, "This is the type of position I would prefer." Show the reader that you really want the job.

- You should take it upon yourself to research the facility to find out all you can. In your cover letter, mention any favorable information (such as the facility's recent achievements). This information will also be effective during the interview process.

- If you know anyone who works at the facility, mention it. However, don't mention the person by name unless you have her permission.

- Make sure you address your letter to the correct person. Call the personnel office and ask for the name of the person handling applications. Use correct spelling and titles (e.g., Mrs., Ms., Mr.).

- Use good-quality paper. Include your name, address, phone number, and e-mail address at the top of the page, centered or in block form.

- Single-space the letter and double-space between paragraphs.

Structurally Speaking

Remember that the facility may receive many applications in a short amount of time, so if your cover letter is too long or tedious, the reader may disregard it altogether. The standard form for a cover letter has three brief paragraphs.

1. *First paragraph.* State the position for which you're applying.
2. *Second paragraph.* Explain your skills and qualifications. Remember that you're also including your resume, so don't be redundant. But emphasize any key skills that are needed for the job.
3. *Third paragraph.* Request an interview. Keep a copy of your cover letter and resume for reference when calling.

E-mail Etiquette

Resumes and cover letters are often submitted to potential employers via e-mail. Understanding basic e-mail etiquette will help you make a good impression. You learned several tips for creating professional e-mail messages in Chapter 2, such as avoiding the use of slang and checking your spelling and grammar. But before you click the "send" button, consider the following additional suggestions.

- Create a separate e-mail account for communicating with prospective employers. Make sure your e-mail address is professional, and consider including your name in the

Edward Hogan, C.M.A
825 Brookefield Ave., Apt. 2
Baltimore, MD 21211
home phone: (410) 555-2121
cell phone: (443) 555-2121
ehogan@email.com

November 18, 2008

Mrs. Sarah Miller
Human Resources Department
St. Sebastian's Children's Hospital
1304 Windy Poplar Ave., Suite 230
Hartford, CT 01385

Dear Mrs. Miller,

I am writing to introduce myself as a recent graduate of the medical assisting program at Greenwood Medical Institute. I feel I am qualified to fill the position of medical assistant that is posted on your Web site.

I graduated Greenwood Medical Institute with a 3.5 GPA and completed an externship at First Care Kids Center. I passed the certification examination and am now a certified medical assistant. While in school, I worked part-time at a daycare center and volunteered at an elementary school. As a result, I have a lot of experience working with children of all ages. I am fully prepared to work in a medical environment that focuses on improving children's health.

I am trained in all of the appropriate medical assisting skills, such as taking accurate notes and handling patient information, explaining procedures to patients, and completing necessary lab tests. I'm ready to put these skills to work for you.

I would be proud to be a part of your medical team. I would like to schedule an appointment with you to go over my resume and learn more about the position. I will call you in a week to set up a meeting. I look forward to meeting with you.

Sincerely,

Edward Hogan

Edward Hogan

A cover letter should be brief but meaningful. It gives the reader a sample of yourself and what you have to offer.

address. An example of a personal e-mail address would be something such as KnicksFan#1@e-mail.com, whereas a professional address would most likely include your name, such as JSmith@e-mail.com.

- You can attach your resume by clicking on the file attachment icon, locating the file, and inserting it. It is always a good idea to open the attachment to make sure you've inserted the correct file before sending it.

- Be concise and to the point. Flowery language will seem pretentious. Remember also that your potential employer may receive many e-mail messages each day, so be courteous by keeping yours brief.
- Avoid adding quotes, colorful borders, or emoticons to your message as these will appear unprofessional.
- Spell out any abbreviations to avoid confusing the recipient.

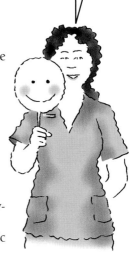

It's fine to use emoticons in your personal e-mails to friends, but avoid including them in your messages to prospective employers.

COMPLETING EMPLOYMENT APPLICATIONS

Some facilities require that you fill out an employment application when interviewing for a job. You may be asked to fill out the application in the office while you wait for the interview, or one may be mailed to you for you to complete beforehand and bring to the interview. Some sites may rely more heavily on the application than on your resume when making their final decision. You should have a generic application already completed to use as a reference when having to complete an application on-site.

Apply Yourself!

Follow these guidelines when completing an application form.

- Read through the entire application before you begin.
- Follow the instructions exactly. Prospective employers notice neatness, erasures, and gaps in the application.
- Answer every question. If a question doesn't apply to you, write "N/A" (not applicable) so the reader knows you didn't simply overlook or avoid the question.
- In the line for wage or salary desired, it's a good idea to write "negotiable" so the employer understands that you're flexible. You may want to find out what the usual salary is for this position before the interview.
- In spaces requesting your reason for leaving your former position, write something positive. "To explore a new career direction" is a positive statement and covers a lot of terrain. If you left because of relocation, schooling, or pregnancy, then say so.
- Use a blue or black pen. Never use a pencil or colored pen (pink, green, purple) as these present an unprofessional image.

Rave Reviews

On the application, you may be asked to list references, such as previous employers or instructors. Consider your options. Whom have you worked with in the past? Was the experience positive? Try to choose people on whom you made a favorable impression. When you have chosen the people you want to use as references, be sure to ask their permission. You may consider including the following people as references:

- instructors
- other medical professionals, such as physicians and nurses
- previous employers
- your externship site coordinator

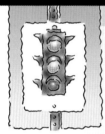

Signs & Signals

HANDLING CALLS FROM PROSPECTIVE EMPLOYERS

Making a good impression starts before the first interview. Here are some tips for handling calls from prospective employers.

- Tell family members or other household members that you're expecting important phone calls.
- Keep a pen and paper by the phone, along with other important information you may need to give, such as your work history or a former employer's phone number.
- Instruct people to take a complete message. Ask them to write down the person's name, phone number, message, and what time the call was received.
- Leave a professional message on your answering machine. Avoid leaving cute or silly messages.

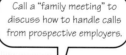

Call a "family meeting" to discuss how to handle calls from prospective employers.

- a physician, registered nurse, or medical assistant from your externship site

Provide a minimum of three references and no more than five. The individuals you select should be able to vouch for your knowledge of medical assisting, skills and abilities, and your previous work experience. Your neighbors, pastor, and relatives may have wonderful things to say about you, but their opinions aren't relevant to your prospective employer, so don't use them as references.

Interviewing

The interview is where you can really shine. It's your chance to show your potential employer who you are and what makes you special. A lot of job candidates look great on paper. They might have all the necessary credentials and experience to do the job well. But if they don't allow their personality to shine through during the interview, they might not get hired. Your potential employer wants to see that you have the personal characteristics to do a good job even during difficult or stressful situations. Make a good impression by showing the interviewer that the quality of your personality characteristics matches the quality of your application or resume.

PREPARATION

Have you ever prepared for a long trip? If so, you know that there are certain things you bring with you and other things you choose to leave behind. Think of the interview as your destination. Which things are you going to bring with you? What do you need to do a good job? Thorough preparation for the interview includes these elements:

- practicing your interviewing skills
- researching the facility where you're applying for a job
- dressing to impress by wearing appropriate professional clothing
- bringing the necessary items with you to the interview

If you enter the interview feeling prepared, you'll project a confident and optimistic attitude to your prospective employer.

Practice, Practice, Practice!

Interviewing is just like any other skill you've learned; it takes practice to get it just right. You can practice for the interview by rehearsing with family or friends. Have someone else act as the interviewer and give him a list of typical questions. (See *Answering Questions.*) Mentally prepare an answer to each question in your head, and practice saying it aloud. Remember though, that the interview is like a conversation, so your responses should sound thoughtful, not robotic.

Have the mock interviewer throw in a tricky question now and then. This will help you react spontaneously and think on your toes. You can also rehearse what you will say in front of a mirror. Practicing first will help the real interview go smoothly, and you'll feel better prepared. Remember that the person who interviews best is usually hired for the job, so pay particular attention to this portion of the application process.

Do Your Research

Part of preparing for the interview is having your facts straight. This means that you should research the facility ahead of time,

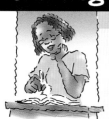

Travelog

IF YOUR RESUME IS LESS THAN SPARKLING

I recently applied for a medical assisting position at a local physician's office. Everything was going smoothly during the interview until my potential employer asked me why I had been fired by my former supervisor. I knew this question might come up, but I was still very nervous about answering it. I took a deep breath and remembered that there is nothing I can do about the past—it's best to be honest. I explained that I was fired because my work was under par. I told her that I realize now what I had been doing incorrectly, and that I should have gone to my former supervisor with more questions. I learned that you have to take a proactive approach to your job, especially when you're unsure of something.

The next day, I got a phone call from the interviewer—I got the job! She said she was impressed that I took ownership of my mistakes and that I was willing to work hard to make changes. Everyone deserves a second chance!

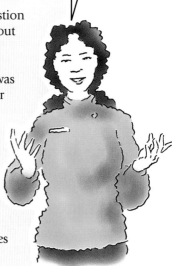

Smooth the rough edges of your employment history by remaining honest and positive during the interview.

so that you're prepared to answer questions and engage the interviewer in discussion. If you're knowledgeable about the facility and job position, you'll feel more confident during the interview. Here are some tips to consider when researching the facility.

- Review your textbooks so that you can ask informed questions about procedures performed at the site. If you'll be interviewing at a specialty practice, be familiar with the types of procedures typically performed in that type of office.
- Think of questions to ask and write them down. Anticipate questions that might be asked of you.
- Find out the name and job title of the interviewer. If it's a difficult name to pronounce, practice saying it aloud.
- Go to the site ahead of time to be sure of its location. Time the trip so you'll be sure to arrive a few minutes early on the day of the interview. Try to take this trip at the same time of day as your actual interview to consider the potential for traffic delays, parking problems, and so forth.

Look the Part

The interview is your chance to impress the interviewer with your personality, skills, and achievements. What better way to wrap up a great package than with the appropriate clothing? If you're dressed professionally, the interviewer will believe that you take this job opportunity seriously and that you will strive to do your best. It's important to pay attention to what your appearance says about you. The general rule is to dress one step above what is required for the job. For positions that require you to wear scrubs, wear appropriate business attire (such as a suit or dress shirt and slacks) to the interview.

Here are some other suggestions to consider when dressing for the interview.

- Avoid overdressing, and make sure your attire is professional and conservative.
- Practice good personal hygiene. If you normally smoke, avoid smoking immediately before the interview. People who don't smoke are often very aware of the odor on someone else's clothes and breath.
- Make sure your breath smells fresh. Chew gum or have a mint before the interview begins. However, don't chew gum during the interview, as this can present an unprofessional image.

- Avoid wearing large jewelry, which can be a distraction.
- If you wear makeup, make sure it is applied tastefully and carefully.
- Avoid wearing strong perfumes or colognes; some people are very sensitive to scents.

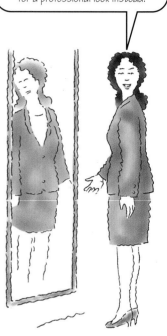

As you prepare for the interview, leave your trendy clothing at home and opt for a professional look instead.

Bring Your Portfolio

A **portfolio** is a folder containing all the information you'll need to impress the interviewer. If you don't have a special folder or briefcase, then a new manila folder will work well, too. A typical portfolio might include the following items:

- pens
- notepads
- your driver's license (or other form of photo identification) and Social Security card
- verification or at least the dates of recent immunizations (hepatitis B, TB test)
- two copies of your resume
- two letters of reference
- copies of any awards or certificates received
- a typed list of at least three references including names, phone numbers, and addresses
- documentation of any special projects or activities in which you've participated

DURING THE INTERVIEW

Keep in mind that the interview isn't just about what's on paper; it's about how you come across in person. Do you have good communication skills? Are you personable and approachable? These skills are just as important to master as your technical skills. Follow these guidelines to make a good impression on the interviewer.

- Make eye contact and smile.
- Shake the interviewer's hand before the interview and introduce yourself properly.
- Display open body language. Keep your arms and legs uncrossed and relaxed. Place your hands in your lap or hold your portfolio.
- Sit with straight posture.

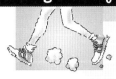

OVERCOMING YOUR ANXIETY

What if you're nervous about the interview? How can you avoid becoming tongue tied and allowing your anxiety to get the better of you?

It's natural to feel nervous before an interview. After all, you've worked very hard for this moment, and you want everything to go smoothly. You can't predict how the interview will go, but there are some things you can do to prepare yourself and handle your nerves.

> Record yourself answering questions during a mock interview. Play it back and see if you need to make any changes to your pacing or enunciation.

On the day of the interview, eat a well-balanced breakfast. A good breakfast gives you energy. Do some stretching or breathing exercises to get the blood circulating in your body. Good circulation increases blood flow to the brain, improving mental functioning. Avoid drinking caffeinated beverages or eating sugary foods as these substances can increase your anxiety level.

Many people stutter, speak too fast, or speak too softly when they're nervous. If you have this problem, practice opening your mouth when you speak and taking the time to enunciate each syllable. Rehearse your answers to common interview questions. Having a good idea of *what* you're going to say allows you to concentrate on *how* you're going to say it. Don't be afraid to pause before answering a question, as this gives you time to think of how to word your response effectively. Remember to breathe and sit up straight. Remind yourself of your accomplishments and skills. If you're feeling relaxed and prepared, your attitude will help you communicate to the interviewer that you're the right person for the job.

Answering Questions

Think positively when answering questions during the interview. Employers will want to see that you take an optimistic approach to your career. Stress your strengths, but be mindful of your weaknesses and how you seek to improve them. Emphasize your skills and accomplishments, but answer all questions truthfully.

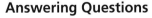

The table below includes a list of common interview questions, their significance, and suggestions to keep in mind when forming your responses. Because these questions are so common, it's a good idea to mentally prepare an answer for each one. Focus on constructing positive responses even when the questions are difficult or probing.

Common Interview Questions		
Question	**Significance**	**Keep in Mind . . .**
What can you tell me about yourself?	The employer wants to get to know who you are, your values, and your experiences.	Who are you? Where are you going? What matters to you?
What are your strengths and weaknesses?	The employer wants to see that you have a firm grasp of who you are as a worker.	Be honest; state weaknesses as opportunities for growth, and explain how you will improve upon them.
Why do you want this position?	The employer wants to understand your motivation for applying for this position.	Emphasize your desire to help others and your interest in the medical field.
Why did you leave your last position?	The employer wants to understand your work history.	Reframe negatives, such as "bad work environment" to "seeking a more positive work environment."
How do you handle pressure?	The employer wants to know if you're able to cope with stress proactively.	Explain techniques you use to handle stress, and how they relate to the position.
Do you work better alone or as a team?	The employer wants to see that you're able and willing to do both.	Explain which you prefer, but *why* you're able to do both.
Who was your best supervisor, and why?	The employer wants to know what you desire in a supervisor.	Include positive remarks, such as "always fair," "supportive," and "encouraging." Avoid comments such as "She gave us long lunch breaks" or "She didn't make us work hard."
How do you handle conflict?	The employer wants to know how well you get along with others.	Explain techniques you use, such as employing good communication skills or always being open to constructive criticism.
How would your classmates describe you?	The employer would like to see how others might see you, and how you see yourself.	Explain some positive characteristics, such as "good student," "team worker," and "helpful," and why a classmate would use them to describe you.
Describe the term *confidentiality* and how you would use it in our office.	The employer wants to see if you understand what confidentiality is and how you would protect it.	What is confidentiality? Why is patient confidentiality important from a legal and ethical viewpoint? Explain how you will uphold confidentiality in the workplace.

Fork in the Road POSITIVE OR PROBLEMATIC?

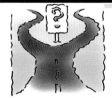

Read the five interview questions and sample responses below. Determine whether each response is effective and positively worded. If it is, write the word "positive." If it isn't, explain why it is problematic and write your own effective response to the question.

1. Question: What are your strengths?
   Response: *I'm empathetic and helpful with patients, and I have excellent technical skills.*

> Your weaknesses can be strengths if you know how to use them to your advantage.

2. Question: What are your weaknesses?
   Response: *I don't have any weaknesses. My instructors told me I was a model student.*

3. Question: Why did you leave your last position?
   Response: *My supervisor was obnoxious and always complained when I was late to work.*

4. Question: How do you handle conflict?
   Response: *I remain levelheaded by taking deep breaths and listening quietly to the other person. Then, I calmly explain my situation and try to reach an agreement.*

5. Question: Do you work better alone or as a member of a team?
   Response: *I try to work alone as often as possible. My coworkers just don't listen to my ideas.*

Asking Questions

The interviewer will usually set aside some time at the end of the interview for you to ask questions. So it's important to have some questions prepared.

It's also a good idea to take notes during the interview so that you can avoid asking questions that have already been answered. Taking notes will also help you form questions in your mind, and asking those questions will clear up any confusion or misunderstandings you may have. As you take notes, focus on the details of the job, salary, and benefits. By the end of your note-taking, you should have several questions for the interviewer.

Here are some common questions you should consider asking.

- What are the responsibilities of the position offered?
- What are the opportunities for future advancement?
- How long is the training or probation period?
- How does the facility feel about continuing education? Is time off offered to employees to upgrade their skills? Does the facility pay for a portion of the expense?
- Is there a job performance or evaluation process?
- What is the benefit package? Will I have access to life insurance? Health insurance? 401(k) or other retirement plan?

Write down the interviewer's answers to your questions for future reference. Make sure the questions you ask are appropriate. Inquiring about details such as time off for vacations implies that you're more interested in being paid to avoid work than in contributing to the work that needs to be done.

Closing

It's important to close the interview by reiterating how important continuing your education is to you. Employers want to hire someone who is willing to put the time and effort into learning new things about the medical field. Discuss the types of continuing education courses you would like to attend. Explain that you realize medicine is always changing, so it's important to stay up to date with the latest developments.

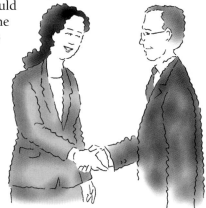

Thank you again for the opportunity to apply for this position.

You can close by thanking the interviewer for the opportunity to apply for the position and shaking her hand. Inquire about the time frame for the decision. Ask if you may call again before the decision date to clear up any questions that the interviewer may have during the decision-making process. Before you leave, obtain the interviewer's business card so you can send a follow-up letter.

Follow-Up

The day after the interview, follow up with a brief thank-you note (see page 210). Express your thanks for the opportunity to be interviewed and restate how interested you are in the job.

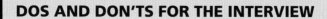

Road Rules DOS AND DON'TS FOR THE INTERVIEW

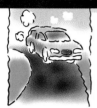

The interview is the most important part of applying for a position. Often, your performance during the interview can make or break your chances of landing the job. Here are some dos and don'ts to keep in mind before, during, and after the interview.

- *Do* practice the interview with a friend or family member. Know how you're going to answer common questions ahead of time.
- *Don't* arrive at the interview unprepared.
- *Do* strive to make a good impression on the interviewer. Display open body language and good communication skills.
- *Do* answer the interviewer's questions honestly and to the best of your ability. Try to put a positive spin on any weaknesses you may have or obstacles you've faced.
- *Don't* criticize past employers, their offices, or your coworkers.
- *Do* ask the interviewer appropriate questions. Show that you're enthusiastic and interested in the position.
- *Don't* ask questions about taking time off for vacations.
- *Do* close the interview by thanking the interviewer for the opportunity to apply for the position.

Good etiquette and an enthusiastic approach may give you an edge over other candidates. Remind the interviewer that you are available for additional questions.

Several days after sending the thank-you note, call the facility. Reintroduce yourself politely and add any new information or ask any questions that may have occurred to you after the interview. Ask if the interviewer has any additional questions for you. Then, thank the interviewer again for the opportunity.

The Search Continues . . .

Suppose several weeks have passed and you haven't heard back from the site where you interviewed. You may need to review your interview performance. Did you impress the interviewer

Maria Sefferin, C.M.A.
11 Jersey Road
Fredericksburg, VA 12345
703-555-0123

Ms. Joan Brown
Office Manager
Middletown Cardiology Consultants
24 Main Street
Williamsburg, VA 12346

October 22, 2008

Dear Ms. Brown:

Thank you for giving me the opportunity to interview for the position of Medical Assistant in your office. I enjoyed meeting you and touring your facility.

I feel I would be an asset to your office for many reasons. I have a strong knowledge of medical terminology, anatomy and physiology, and cardiac diseases. I have solid clinical and administrative skills. I believe that this position will offer me an opportunity to use the education and training that I have received in my medical assisting courses.

I am very interested in this position. This is the type of career opportunity that I had hoped to find. If you have any questions, please feel free to call me at 703-555-0123.

Sincerely,

Maria Sefferin, C.M.A.

Follow up after an interview with a brief thank-you note.

with your communication and relational skills? Were those or other skills lacking in your manner or on your resume? Reevaluate what you said during the interview and think about how you can improve your performance during future interviews.

WHY WASN'T I HIRED?

Here are some common reasons why a candidate isn't hired:

- poor personal appearance
- lack of purpose or direction
- inappropriate demeanor (overly enthusiastic or aggressive)
- lack of tact or diplomacy
- failure to make eye contact
- inappropriate humor
- poorly completed or messy application and resume
- overemphasis on the need for time off or a higher salary

Other factors that may impact a candidate's ability to get a job include credit scores and criminal background checks. For example, with your consent, potential employers may obtain information about your credit history. If you're applying for a position that involves the handling of money (such as that of a medical billing specialist), low credit scores may make it more difficult for you to get the job. Likewise, a criminal conviction can also harm a candidate's chances of working in health care. However, this decision may be made on a case-by-case basis, depending on the nature of the crime.

It's extremely important to report any previous criminal convictions on your job application. Although a conviction in itself may not disqualify you for the job, lying on your job application certainly will!

IS THE JOB SEARCH TAKING TOO LONG?

The average job search takes six months or longer. If you feel that your job search is taking too long, then consider the following questions.

- Are you conducting your job search half-heartedly?
- Does your resume need to be critiqued or updated?
- Have you tried using different methods or resources for your job search?
- Are you keeping a journal of your job search activity?
- Do you need more interview practice?

Ask The Professional | HOW CAN I SPEED UP MY JOB SEARCH?

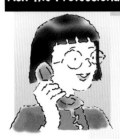

Q: *My job search seems to be taking a long time. Is there anything I can do to help speed up the process?*

A: After you send your resume and cover letter or attend a job interview, it may seem as though your only option is to wait for the phone to ring. But there are several ways you can be proactive and ensure that your job search keeps moving at a steady pace.

First, remember to follow up each interview by sending a thank-you note and calling the employment site. When you follow up, briefly remind the interviewer who you are and reiterate your interest in the position. Sometimes, a site will get so many applicants that you have to find a way to stand out from the crowd.

Next, consider how you may come across during an interview. Is your demeanor open and friendly? Are you able to convey your enthusiasm for the job to potential employers? Do you project a professional manner during interviews? Work on honing your interview skills with a friend or colleague, and ask for his opinion.

Finally, continue searching for additional job opportunities while you're awaiting an answer from a potential employer. It never hurts to have a "plan B" already in motion just in case an opportunity falls through. By keeping your options open, you might even have to choose between more than one job offer!

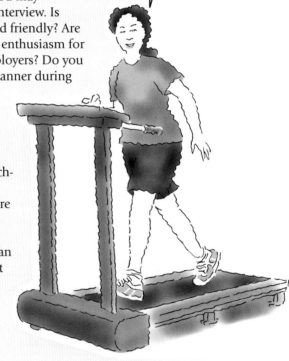

Does it feel like you've been working hard but your job search just isn't going anywhere? Adjust your approach and keep trying!

- Is it time to consider a temporary agency or a part-time position?
- Do you need to acquire or improve a specific skill?

Before You Accept a Position

Before you decide to accept a position, ask yourself the following questions.

- Am I qualified for the position?
- Will I be proud to say I work there?
- How far is the job from home?
- Are there opportunities for advancement?
- Will I earn enough to pay my bills?
- What will my take-home pay be after taxes (including federal, state, and local taxes, along with other deductions)?
- Are benefits included? Does the company offer health insurance and a 401(k) plan?
- Do I need to seek advice from one of my instructors, the career services director at school, or my family and close friends?
- Is the employer asking me to make a rushed decision? If so, why?
- Will it be easy to get along with the other staff members I met? Will the position be a good fit for me from a personality perspective?

Keep in mind that certain details, such as the position's salary and benefits, may be negotiable. If you'd like to accept a position but are worried that the salary or benefits package won't meet your needs, discuss your concerns with the employer. Research typical salaries for the position in your area, being careful to make adjustments for your levels of training and experience. Use this information to back up any requests you make for increases in salary or benefits. By maintaining a positive and professional attitude during these negotiations, the employer will be more likely to work with you to reach a solution that is satisfactory for both parties involved.

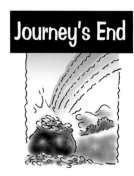

Journey's End

- You may be faced with obstacles to employment as a medical assistant, such as a lack of experience, gaps in your employment, or being fired from a previous job. Maintaining a positive attitude is one way to overcome these obstacles.

- Set goals for yourself by determining your ideal job. Think about the many elements that make up each job and describe the type of position you'd like to find. Consider the type of facility where you'd like to work, which duties you'd like to perform, and what your ideal working hours would be.

- Set realistic career goals for yourself by researching estimated industry growth and typical salaries for medical assistants. In terms of position and income, decide where you'd like to be in the next two to five years.

- Several basic job search methods include networking with contacts in the medical field, visiting your school's career placement office, and searching for job advertisements online. The key to conducting a successful job search is using all the resources available to you.

- Creating effective resumes and cover letters will let employers know that you are a professional and that you take your work seriously.

- Using effective communication skills and interview techniques will make a good impression on potential employers and help you land the job. Often, the candidate who interviews best is the one who is offered the position.

- Before accepting or declining a job offer, consider factors such as possible opportunity for advancement, salary and benefits, office environment, and the length of your commute.

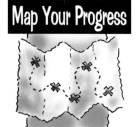

Map Your Progress

Answer the following multiple-choice questions.

1. Which of the following is *not* a good reason to provide for gaps in your employment?
   a. schooling
   b. relocation
   c. long commute
   d. pregnancy

2. Which of the following individuals would make the *best* reference?
   a. best friend
   b. rabbi

    c. former supervisor
    d. karate instructor

3. What information should you include on your resume?
    a. recommendations from instructors, strengths and weaknesses, and salary requirements
    b. education, skills, and appropriate affiliations or volunteer work
    c. grades, references, and hobbies and personal interests outside of work
    d. all of the above

4. A *chronological* resume:
    a. works well for those who recently graduated or who are reentering the workforce after a significant absence.
    b. focuses on your skills and qualifications rather than on your employment history.
    c. is preferred by employers seeking to fill medical assisting positions.
    d. lists your previous positions (including your job title and key responsibilities) in order by date.

5. Why should you know something about the employment site before the interview?
    a. so you can ask appropriate questions
    b. so you can send a thank-you note
    c. so you know more than the interviewer
    d. so you can skip the interview

6. Why is the medical assisting profession expected to grow in coming years?
    a. There are fewer people going into the medical field.
    b. The population is aging.
    c. The country is experiencing economic growth.
    d. There are fewer physicians.

7. Which of the following is *not* an appropriate question to ask during a job interview?
    a. How many vacation days do employees get each year?
    b. What is the benefit package offered for the position?
    c. Does the facility help cover the costs of continuing education?
    d. What are the opportunities for future advancement?

8. A *portfolio* is:
    a. a file kept by your academic advisor that includes your school transcripts.
    b. a manila envelope containing the resources you've gathered during your job search.

    c. a folder containing all the information you'll need to impress the interviewer.
    d. none of the above

9. How long does the average job search take?
    a. one month
    b. two months
    c. four months
    d. six months

10. What might keep you from getting a job?
    a. poor personal appearance
    b. a sloppy or incomplete job application
    c. an overly aggressive attitude
    d. all of the above

Chapter 7

THE JOURNEY CONTINUES: CAREER SUCCESS AND ADVANCEMENT

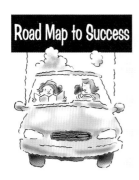

Road Map to Success

- Explain the importance of sound technical and soft skills to success in your job

- Identify ways to abide by medical assisting standards of ethics and conduct

- Identify three ways in which you can show interest in your job and your employer

- List the benefits of finding a mentor and building rapport with experienced coworkers

- Describe how you can be a respectful and dependable coworker

- Explain why it's important for health care professionals to continue their education and keep up with the latest trends in health care and medicine

- Explain how renewing your certification and joining a professional organization will help you expand your career opportunities

- Identify your career goals and develop a plan for achieving them

- List the elements to consider when deciding whether to leave a job and seek new opportunities

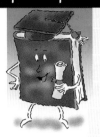

Chapter Competencies

- Conduct work within scope of education, training, and ability (ABHES 1.i.)

- Be cognizant of ethical boundaries (ABHES 1.d.)

- Perform within legal and ethical boundaries (CAAHEP 3.c.2.b.)

- Exhibit initiative (ABHES 1.e.)

- Adapt to change (ABHES 1.f.)

- Project a positive attitude (ABHES 1.a.)

- Be a "team player" (ABHES 1.c.)

- Evidence a responsible attitude (ABHES 1.g.)

- Be courteous and diplomatic (ABHES 1.h.)

Succeeding in your job is the first step toward advancing in your career. In this chapter, you'll discover how to apply the skills, ethical guidelines, and professional behaviors you've learned in this book toward your first medical assisting job. You'll also learn how to excel as a medical assistant and advance in your career through:

- continuing your education
- maintaining your certification
- joining an appropriate professional organization

Because achieving success in your career sometimes involves leaving a position and seeking new opportunities, you'll also read about when to keep and when to leave a job.

You've Got Skills!

Everyone has certain skills. The bus driver who takes you to and from work each day most likely has good driving skills. A ship's captain knows how to sail from one shore to another. And a conductor is able to keep the train on the right track. In short, the better your medical assisting skills are, the better you will be at your job and the more likely you will advance in your career.

As you learned from previous chapters, you are responsible for incorporating two kinds of skills into your work as a medical assistant:

- technical skills, or the performance of patient care skills and the proper use of equipment and technology

- soft skills, or the use of effective communication, interpersonal skills, and professional behavior

> Technical skills are the "nuts and bolts" of medical assisting. Mastering these skills will give you the confidence you need to do your job well.

By now, you've probably developed these skills as a student and throughout your externship, but perfecting them will take practice and dedication. Your job will provide you with daily opportunities to use your skills and fine-tune them. Each time you work with a patient or staff member, you are using a skill that you've learned. You may also have the opportunity to share these skills when you work as a team member or when you explain something to a new coworker. And, as technology and science progress and develop, you will learn new skills that will improve the care you provide to patients.

TECHNICAL SKILLS

Technical skills are the "nuts and bolts" of medical assisting. These skills allow you to use medical equipment properly and perform basic tasks related to patient care.

Rules to Work By

Any time you're working with medical equipment or materials, make sure that you're using them properly. Remember, though, that the proper technique you learned inside the classroom may be different from what is expected of you on the job. So, it's important to be flexible and willing to adapt your technique to the office's policies and procedures.

Although techniques can vary depending on the medical office in which you're working, some general guidelines apply to all situations. When performing technical skills, ask yourself:

- Are the materials/equipment clean and sterile?
- Am I using the appropriate materials/equipment for the task?
- Are any parts of the materials/equipment damaged, broken, or missing?
- Am I following proper protocol?
- Am I taking proper safety precautions to protect myself and the patient?

If you're having doubts about your ability to perform a task, stop and ask someone to help you. It's always better to take a step back, ask a question, or ask for assistance than to jeopardize the health and safety of a patient.

Learn by Observation

If you're having trouble perfecting a skill, you can learn more by observing other medical professionals. You can ask questions and apply what you've learned to your own technique. You'll also have the opportunity to develop your technique with patients every day, so your skills will naturally improve over time.

SOFT SKILLS

Your job as a medical professional involves more than simply performing skills and caring for patients' physical problems. It also includes soft skills, or behaving professionally and providing patients with genuine support and compassion as they work through their treatment and healing.

You've learned about soft skills in previous chapters, so the list below should seem familiar. You have likely practiced these skills in the classroom and during your externship. Keep in mind that soft skills include the following.

- *Communication skills* include verbal and nonverbal messages. What you say and how you say it influences others' perceptions of you and the medical office, so you should strive to communicate positively and effectively.

- *Customer service* refers to the quality of health care provided to patients. You should always strive to meet patients' needs and ensure patient satisfaction by building trust and establishing a good rapport.

- *Empathy* is the ability to understand what someone else is feeling. Your empathy for patients lets them know that you care about their needs and how they're feeling, which can result in increased trust and better communication.

- *Impartiality* is the ability to treat all patients equally, with the same care and concern. Every patient has the right to equal treatment.

- *Courtesy* should be given to every patient who enters the office. Patients must be treated respectfully and with gracious manners.

- *Diplomacy and tact* help you effectively manage people with sensitivity and genuine concern. The right word at the right moment can relieve a potentially tense situation.

Travelog

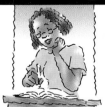

LEADER OR BOSS?

I was new on the job and eager to make a positive impact on my fellow coworkers. During team meetings, I would readily state my opinion and encourage others to agree with me. If someone had a different viewpoint, I would quickly prove him wrong. I thought I was being a great leader by being forceful and direct.

One day, one of my coworkers came to me with a worried expression on her face. She told me that everyone liked how enthusiastic I was about my job, but that I never gave anyone else a chance to speak during discussions. I knew she was right. Even though I was friendly and talkative, none of the other staff members seemed happy to work with me. I realized that by coming on like a bulldozer, I had knocked over everyone else! I guess I was worried that I wouldn't have what it takes to be a good medical assistant, so I tried to overcompensate by being a "leader." Now I understand that a real leader listens to others' viewpoints instead of only hearing her own.

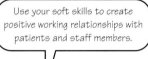

Use your soft skills to create positive working relationships with patients and staff members.

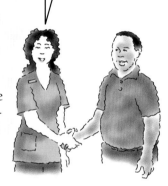

New Job Jitters

So you have a great new job, but maybe you're still feeling apprehensive or shy. After all, you're in a new environment with new people, and there is so much to learn and take in all at once. It's best to be honest with yourself and others. If you're feeling overwhelmed, then tell someone. Maybe your supervisor is explaining something too quickly, or the information is too detailed and you need a moment to reflect. These and other stressors are inherent to any new job. Here are some tips for handling these situations.

- Take a note pad and pen everywhere with you. The first week or so of a new job, you'll be given a lot of new information, and some of it may not be in written form for you. If you think you'll forget it, then write it down!

- When you meet a coworker for the first time, shake hands and introduce yourself. Tell the person that you're a new employee, and it may take some time to adjust, but that you're looking forward to working with him or her.

- Ask questions! There is an entire staff that has the experience and skills to answer your questions, so if you don't know or aren't sure, ask someone!
- Tell someone if you don't understand something or need further clarification.
- Keep a positive attitude. Change can be stressful, but also rewarding. You've got a great new job and you've reached many of your goals already! Keep in mind that you won't be the "newbie" for very long; eventually, you'll be comfortable enough to assist other new employees.

Ethics and Conduct in the Workplace

What is right? What is wrong? How can we tell the two apart? Sometimes, the lines between right and wrong aren't so clear.

Rules and laws tell us explicitly what we can and can't do. You follow rules every day. For example, when you drive a car, pay a bill, or wait in line, you are adhering to rules and laws that are in place to keep you safe and maintain order. Rules and laws are important to follow because they support the principles upheld by our society.

As a medical assistant, you will adhere to the principles that govern the medical community. As you learned in Chapter 1, these principles are called ethics, and they establish the code of moral and ethical conduct that governs the behavior of medical professionals.

AAMA MEDICAL ASSISTANT CODE OF ETHICS

By now, you probably feel that you've developed a solid understanding of the basic principles that a medical assistant should seek to uphold. Honesty, hard work, and compassion for others are just a few of the characteristics that will keep you on the right track in your career. But you may still be wondering exactly what or who determines ethical conduct for medical assistants.

The American Association of Medical Assistants (AAMA) has created a set of five principles of ethical and moral conduct that all medical assistants must follow. The code states that medical assistants should always strive to:

- provide services with respect for human dignity
- protect patient confidentiality (except when required by law to reveal private information)

- uphold the honor and high principles of the medical assisting profession
- improve knowledge and skills continually for the benefit of patients and the health care team
- participate in community service activities that promote the health and well-being of the general public

AAMA MEDICAL ASSISTANT CREED

The AAMA has also written a creed for medical assistants. A creed is a system of principles or beliefs that a group of people chooses to follow. As a medical assistant who continually strives to uphold the principles of the profession, you should know the AAMA Medical Assistant Creed and understand how its principles seek to improve the medical community and the care provided to patients. The creed is:

- I believe in the principles and purposes of the medical profession.
- I seek to be more effective.
- I aspire to render greater service.
- I protect the confidence entrusted to me.
- I am dedicated to the care and well-being of all people.
- I am loyal to my employer.
- I am true to the ethics of my profession.
- I am strengthened by compassion, courage, and faith.

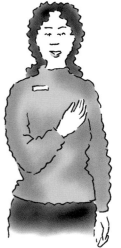

When you recite the AAMA Medical Assistant Creed, you are pledging your allegiance to patients and the medical community.

YOU CAN'T HAVE ONE WITHOUT THE OTHER

Ethical conduct can be boiled down to two simple characteristics: honesty and integrity. A medical assistant with integrity respects the ethical standards of the profession and does his best to abide by these standards at all times. You have the power to affect the health of patients, and that is not a responsibility to be taken lightly. The quality of the care you provide should reflect your level of integrity.

Honesty is a characteristic that goes hand in hand with integrity. If you're honest in everything you do and say, then you have integrity, because you acknowledge that patients and staff members have a right to the truth. Having honesty and integrity also means that you:

- admit to mistakes and try to correct them
- take full responsibility for your actions

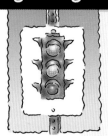

Signs & Signals APPLYING THE PRINCIPLES

Principles are the driving force behind all your actions, good and bad. And how you act shows others what you value. But how do you use principles in day-to-day life as a medical assistant? Here are some tips to help you incorporate the AAMA's principles into your daily tasks in the medical office:

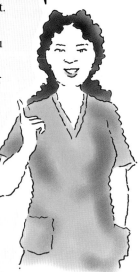

Following HIPAA rules is another way to ensure that you're abiding by appropriate legal and ethical guidelines.

- Treat the patient, not the disease. Caring for patients as individuals with feelings and needs shows them that you value their right to dignity and respect.

- Learn new techniques and skills, and incorporate them into your work. This shows patients that you strive to provide them with the best care.

- Respect patients' right to privacy by protecting their medical records and private health information. Doing so shows that you're trustworthy.

- Treat all patients equally, with the same courtesy and fairness. Patients will understand that you value them and their health concerns.

- Work cooperatively with staff and physicians. This shows your coworkers that you value harmonious relationships.

- Follow all policies and procedures. This lets patients know that you have their safety in mind and their best interests at heart.

- know your professional limits
- never exaggerate, lie, or make false claims

Keep in mind that, when you display honesty and integrity, you'll inspire confidence and trust in your employer, which can lead to success in your job and additional career opportunities in the future.

SURVEY YOUR TERRAIN

As a medical assistant, you have a duty to provide the best possible care to patients. Providing reliable health care involves making decisions regarding which actions will yield the best results in any given situation. Sometimes, a task or decision will exceed the level of your training or abilities. That is, it may fall outside your **scope of practice** as a medical assistant. In these situations, it's important to stop and ask for help from the physician or another qualified health care professional. Attempting to perform a task that you aren't trained or qualified to do can result in legal and ethical consequences for you and the physician.

The duties of a medical assistant are divided into two categories:

- administrative duties
- clinical duties

Your duties as a medical assistant will depend, in part, on the type of medical practice in which you work. For example, medical assistants who work in family practice offices often do a lot of clinical work. However, if you work in a psychiatric practice, you will probably be required to perform more administrative tasks. State law also has a role in determining which tasks you're legally able to perform. This is because laws governing the scope of practice for medical assistants vary from state to state.

The table below provides a list of the types of tasks you may be expected to perform in the medical office.

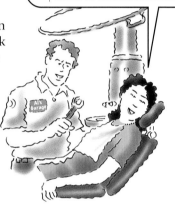

You wouldn't want your mechanic to pull your tooth, would you? Only perform tasks that are within the scope of practice for medical assistants.

Duties of a Medical Assistant

Administrative Duties	Clinical Duties
• managing and maintaining the waiting room, office, and examining rooms • handling phone calls • using written and oral communication skills • maintaining medical records • bookkeeping • scheduling appointments • ensuring good public relations • maintaining office supplies • screening sales representatives • coding and filing insurance forms • processing the payroll • arranging patient hospitalizations • sorting and filing mail • instructing new patients about office hours and relevant office policies • completing medical transcriptions	• preparing patients for examinations and treatments • assisting the physician and other staff members with procedures • preparing and sterilizing instruments • completing electrocardiograms • applying Holter monitors • obtaining medical histories • administering medications and immunizations • obtaining vital signs (blood pressure, pulse, temperature, respirations) • documenting in patients' medical records • performing eye and ear irrigations • recognizing and treating medical emergencies • providing patient education

HANDLING MISTAKES

Following all policies and procedures and working within your scope of practice will decrease the risk of accidents. Even so, mistakes can happen. Everyone, including our mentors, will make mistakes from time to time, so don't be too hard on yourself when they occur. Focus on learning from your mistakes and think about how you can avoid them in the future. Ask yourself, "What happened, and what could I do differently next time?"

I Made a Mistake . . . Now What?

It's your responsibility to notify your supervisor immediately about any mistakes you make on the job. Mistakes that can affect the health of a patient, such as medication errors, must be addressed immediately. In these situations, the physician will know the appropriate steps to take.

However, mistakes don't always involve the potential for physical harm to a patient or staff member. For example, you may make a mistake while carrying out coding or billing tasks. These types of errors, if they aren't corrected, could lead to legal consequences for the physician.

Regardless of the nature of the mistake, your first priority should be to inform your supervisor so the error can be remedied.

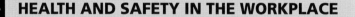

Road Rules **HEALTH AND SAFETY IN THE WORKPLACE**

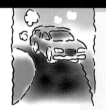

It's true that mistakes can happen in the medical office. But the good news is that there are rules and regulations in place to protect patients and employees. The Occupational Safety and Health Administration (OSHA) is a federal agency that regulates health and safety concerns in the workplace. Many rules under OSHA will affect your job as a medical assistant. Examples include rules for:

- protection from bloodborne pathogens
- use of personal protective equipment, such as disposable gloves and face masks
- tuberculosis prevention
- biohazardous waste disposal

These rules and other guidelines can be found on the OSHA website (www.osha.gov). It's important to be familiar with the regulations that apply to the medical office where you work. Noncompliance with OSHA regulations can result in fines and, in some cases, closure of the health care organization.

Mistakes may not be readily evident. It's important to own up to your mistakes.

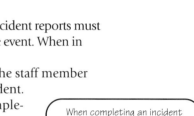

Being honest about your mistakes is the first step toward fixing them.

When Something Happens . . .

When certain mistakes occur, an **incident report** must be completed to document the event. An incident report is a written account of any negative patient, visitor, or staff event, such as:

- all medication errors
- all patient, employee, and visitor falls
- drawing blood from the wrong patient
- mislabeling of blood tubes or specimens
- employee needlesticks
- injuries sustained at the workplace

Such events may be minor or life threatening. Incident reports must be completed even if no injury resulted from the event. When in doubt, always complete an incident report.

An incident report must be completed by the staff member involved in or present at the scene of the incident. The report is reviewed by a supervisor for completion and accuracy and is then sent to the office manager or physician. If a mistake involves a patient, the physician should assess the patient's condition and document the findings on the incident report.

When completing an incident report, remember to include just the facts! Avoid drawing your own conclusions about the event.

Follow these guidelines when filling out an incident report.

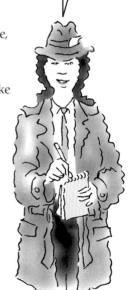

- State only the facts, but be specific. Don't exaggerate, draw conclusions, or summarize the event.
- Write legibly and sign your name legibly.
- Complete the form in a timely fashion. For the sake of accuracy, incident reports should be completed within 24 hours of the event.
- Do not leave any blank spaces on the form. If a particular section of the form doesn't apply, write N/A (not applicable).
- Never photocopy an incident report for your own personal record. This violates patients' confidentiality rights.
- Never place the incident report in the patient's chart or document in the patient's chart that an incident report was completed. For legal reasons, only document the event in the patient's chart.

INCIDENT REPORT FORM
PRIVILEGED & CONFIDENTIAL

Patient Stamp

☐ Inpatient ☐ Outpatient ☐ Visitor ☐ Volunteer ☐ Other   *NOT A PART OF THE MEDICAL RECORD–FORWARD TO RISK MANAGER WITHIN 72 HOURS*

Name		Age	Sex	Admit Date	Location of Incident	Room #
Diagnosis	Date of Incident	Time ____ AM/PM		Date of Report	Person Reporting & Title (print)	

CONDITION BEFORE INCIDENT
☐ Alert ☐ Disoriented ☐ Unconscious ☐ Agitated
☐ Confused ☐ Sedated ☐ Uncooperative ☐ Other

Activity Orders
☐ Adib ☐ BRP ☐ BRP c help
☐ With assist ☐ CBR
☐ Up in chair ☐ BSC

Signature

INCIDENT (please check all items that apply)
FALLS

FALLS	PREFALL FACTORS	RESTRAINTS	RISK CONDITIONS	CURRENT MEDICATIONS
☐ Fall from Bed	☐ Bed Up	Restraints Ordered ☐ Y ☐ N	☐ Weakness ☐ Decreased Mobility	☐ None
☐ Fall from Chair	☐ Bed Down	Restraints in Use ☐ Y ☐ N	☐ Confusion	☐ NTG ☐ Diuretics
☐ Fall from Bedside Commode	☐ Brake On ☐ Y ☐ N	Type: ☐ Vest ☐ Wrist ☐ Ankle	☐ Neuro/ortho diagnosis	☐ Cathartic preps/enemas
☐ Fall from Stretcher	☐ Not working	☐ Secured Mittens	☐ Cardiovascular diagnosis	☐ Antihypertensives
☐ Fall from Wheelchair		☐ Tied ☐ Untied by:	☐ Inpaired Vision	☐ Antiseizure
☐ Fall from Toilet	☐ Siderails Down	____ Staff	☐ History of Syncope	☐ Antidepressants
☐ Fall while Ambulatory	____ 2 Up	____ Patient	☐ Poor Nutritional Status	☐ Antiemetics
☐ Other_____	____ 3 Up	____ Family/S.O.	☐ Incontinence	☐ Antipsychotics
	____ 4 Up		☐ History of fall last 6 months	☐ Analgesics/Hypnotics
	____ Climbed Out	Call light in reach ☐ Y ☐ N	Safety Education given prior to fall:	☐ Narcotics
		Fall follow-up program initiated	☐ None ☐ Patient ☐ Family/S.O.	☐ Cardiovascular
		prior to fall ☐ Y ☐ N		

Environment: ☐ Floor wet ☐ Y ☐ N ☐ Free from obstacles ☐ Y ☐ N Describe: _____
☐ Night light on ☐ Y ☐ N ☐ N/A ☐ Objects not in reach-searching for _____

MEDICATION VARIANCE, Including IV & Blood Product(s)		PROCEDURE VARIANCE		MISCELLANEOUS
☐ Incorrect Pt. Identification	☐ Incorrect IV Solution	☐ Record Error ☐ Transcription	☐ Documentation Error	☐ AMA/Elopement
☐ Incorrect Dosage	☐ Incorrect IV Rate	☐ Incorrect Pt. Identification	☐ Consent Variance	☐ Admitted c Pressure Sore
☐ Incorrect Route	☐ Incorrect Count/Missing Med	☐ Omitted Treatment	☐ Improper Prep of Pt.	☐ Damaged/Lost Teeth/ Denture
☐ Incorrect Time	☐ Topical Substance Reaction, including Tape	☐ Delayed Treatment	☐ NPO Violated	☐ Injury During Transport
☐ Incorrect Med Given	☐ Allergy Not Documented	☐ Omitted Diagnostic/Lab	☐ Radiation/Toxic Chemical Exposure	☐ Self Inflicted Injury/Suicide
☐ Incorrect Med Dispensed	☐ Contrast Reaction/Complication	☐ Delayed Diagnostic/Lab	☐ X-ray Interpretation Discrepancy	☐ Malpositioning/Incorrect Body Alignment
☐ Med Omitted	☐ Medication Past Due 1 hour or more	☐ Traumatic Venipuncture	☐ Airway/Intubation Problem	☐ Pt. Self Extubation
☐ Med Transcription Error	☐ Other_____	☐ Break in Sterile Technique	☐ Incorrect Level of Heat/Cold Applied	☐ Tube/IV Catheter Out
☐ Incorrect Blood Given		☐ Incorrect Surgical Count–Sponge	☐ Incorrect Procedure/Treatment	☐ Accidental Strking Against an Object
☐ Pharmacy Notified		☐ Incorrect Surgical Count–Needle	☐ Unordered Procedure/Treatment	☐ Fainted
☐ Infiltration		☐ Incorrect Surgical Count–Instrument	☐ Equip./Product Malfunction	☐ Pt. Dissatisfied/Pt. Threatened Law Suit
☐ Blood Reaction		☐ Retained Foreign Body	☐ User Error	☐ Transfer to Critical Care p incident
☐ Med Reaction		☐ Other: _____	☐ Equipment Unavailable	☐ Behavior Out of Norm.
		_____		☐ Other: _____

INJURY (please check all items that apply) All serious/significant injuries must be described on reverse side
PROCEDURE/LABOR & DELIVERY/NURSERY

SERIOUS	SIGNIFICANT	SUPERFICIAL	
☐ None	☐ None	☐ None	☐ Newborn with apparent Cerebral dysfunction
☐ Spinal Cord Injury	☐ Major Infiltration	☐ Unknown	☐ Newborn with APGAR of four (4) or less at five (5) minutes
☐ Injury to Nerves	☐ Hospital Acquired Decubiti	☐ Abrasion	☐ Newborn with serious birth trauma
☐ Brain Injury	☐ Burn	☐ Bruising	☐ Precipitous Delivery
☐ Surgery to Wrong Pt.	☐ Fracture	☐ Blister/Skin Tear	☐ Unattended Delivery
☐ Incorrect Surgical Procedure	☐ Sprain/Strain Joint/Muscle	☐ Skin Prick	**MEDICAL DEVICE/EQUIPMENT RELATED**
☐ Shock	☐ Injury to Blood Vessel	☐ Laceration	Equipment involved: _____
☐ Trauma Causing Internal Injury	☐ Dislocation of Joint	☐ Rash/Hives	Manufacturer: _____
☐ Hemorrhage	☐ Open Wound Needing Medical Care	☐ Other:	Serial #: _____
☐ Death	☐ Adverse Effect Due to Med/Anesthesia/Transfusion		Asset #: _____
☐ Unscheduled Return to OR	☐ Adverse Effect Due to Exposure to Toxic Chemical	_____	Biomedical Dept. Notified: _____ Date
☐ Other:	☐ Complication Due to Mechanical Device	_____	Tagged & Removed from Service: _____ Date/Time
	☐ Prolongation of Hospital Stay	_____	**Maintain all components of device such as connectors, adaptors, tubings, etc. Document all readings/settings.**
	☐ Anoxia/Respiratory Distress		
	☐ Cancellation of or after induction of anesthesia		**DO NOT ADJUST OR CLEAR ANY READINGS.**

AMA FOLLOW-UP

Reason for leaving: _____
Patient admitted <24 hours ☐ Yes ☐ No
Patient/S.O. Teaching: ☐ Completed ☐ Partial ☐ None ☐ Patient Uncooperative

Although every medical office has its own form, most incident reports require similar data.

Description of event: _____
_____
_____
_____
_____
_____
_____
_____
_____
_____
_____
_____
_____
_____
_____
_____
_____

Physician notified: ☐ Yes   ☐ No   Name of Physician (print): _____
Physician Remarks: _____
_____
_____
_____
_____
_____
_____
_____

Physician Signature	Date

Supervisor/Manager Investigation/Follow-up Action: _____
_____
_____
_____
_____
_____
_____

Supervisor/Manager Signature	Date

Witness: Name (print)	Department/Shift	Address	Phone

Risk Manager Signature	Date

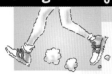

Running Smoothly

KEEPING IT PROFESSIONAL

What if a patient misinterprets your friendliness as flirtation?

Most patients will appreciate a friendly and cheerful attitude. But sometimes, people can mistake a friendly touch or kind gesture as something more. If you feel that a patient has misinterpreted something you've said or done, then explain what you meant. If the person persists, then firmly state that your relationship must remain professional. Remaining firmly within the legal and ethical boundaries of your position will help you provide the best possible health care to patients.

> Friendliness can sometimes be mistaken for flirtation, but don't let that keep you from reaching out when you feel a patient needs therapeutic touch.

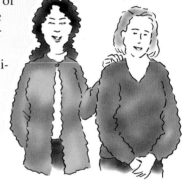

ADHERING TO BOUNDARIES

Sometimes, a patient or coworker can cross an ethical or legal boundary. In these situations, it's your duty to take a step back and consider what to do. For example, if you witness a coworker gossiping about a patient's illness, then you have an obligation to address the situation. You may need to confront your coworker about her inappropriate behavior, or, if that discussion fails to bring about any change, notify your supervisor.

It's also necessary to be aware of boundaries in your relationships with patients. As you read in Chapter 3, keeping a professional distance from patients helps you remain objective and provide better care. Although it's important to be compassionate and caring, your involvement with patients should always remain at a professional level.

Put Your Heart into It

How can you show interest in your job—that it's more than just a 9 to 5 commitment? Showing initiative is the name of the game. Showing initiative lets others know that you care about the workplace and the patients, and that you want to do a good job. Here are ways in which you can show initiative around the office.

- *Going the extra mile.* Helping out wherever necessary, without being asked to, shows that you care about getting the job done. Remember though, that you should only complete those tasks that fall within your scope of practice.
- *Keeping a notebook.* Making a list of supplies and things that are needed in the office will help you keep track of materials. It will also show your employer that you're organized and prepared.
- *Assuming new responsibilities.* Taking on new tasks when you're ready to do so will show your employer that you enjoy a challenge and are willing to work hard.
- *Asking for feedback.* Inquiring about your job performance and accepting constructive criticism will tell your employer that you value the quality of work that you do.
- *Finding a mentor.* Identifying a qualified person to mentor, or guide, you shows your employer that you value experience and enjoy working with and learning from others.
- *Building rapport with experienced coworkers.* Friendliness and teamwork keep the office running smoothly and show patients that your goal is to create harmonious interactions.

Being a Respectful and Dependable Coworker

Close your eyes and imagine a small, still body of water. If you throw a pebble into the water, what happens? The pebble sends ripples through the water, changing its motion and direction. The greater the impact on the water, the more dynamic and far-reaching the change will be.

As a medical assistant, you're very much like that pebble. You have the ability to influence the entire medical team. So how do you send positive ripples through the office? One way is by being a respectful and dependable coworker.

A good coworker is a good medical assistant. She remembers that her actions and decisions affect others. She adheres to the principles set forth by the AAMA and strives to provide the very best care for patients. In short, a good coworker is someone you enjoy working with because she makes the medical office a more positive and productive place to be.

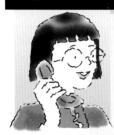

Ask The Professional | FINDING A MENTOR

Q: *How can I find a mentor, and why is having a mentor important?*

A: A mentor can be a fellow coworker, a former instructor, or another member of the medical community who can provide you with guidance as you begin your career. Remember that not everyone makes a good mentor; your mentor should be a more experienced professional with whom you've built a good relationship.

One option for finding a mentor is to contact a professional association, such as the AAMA. If you're a member of the AAMA, you can visit their website and click on "Member Center" at the top of the page. Next, click on "Find a Mentor" in the drop-down menu to learn how you can find a mentor.

You may also consider contacting your academic advisor and asking if your school has a mentoring program in place. If so, a former student from the school can make an excellent mentor.

Those first few months on the job are a time of change and transition, so it's a good idea to have a mentor who can support you in your efforts. The purpose of your new mentor is not unlike that of your externship mentor; both are there to help you refine and improve your skills. After your externship ends, it's just as important to continue learning and improving your skills!

Consider your former coworkers or peers and the positive characteristics they possessed. What characteristics define the ideal coworker? In general, a good coworker is:

- *Cooperative.* He knows how to be a team player and is willing to listen to and support others. He understands that sometimes two heads are better than one!

- *Consistent.* He shows up to work on time every day because he values the hard work and time that others put in and wants to contribute his best effort to reach a common goal.

- *Fair.* He doesn't abuse his sick days and vacation time and tries to avoid scheduling these days during the busiest times of the year. He knows that he has an obligation to be there for his coworkers and patients.

- *Helpful.* He offers his assistance to patients and coworkers without hesitation, unless the tasks fall outside his scope of practice.
- *Dedicated.* He is willing to assume new responsibilities and meets challenges with a positive attitude.
- *Diplomatic.* He stays out of office politics and makes an effort to get along with his coworkers.

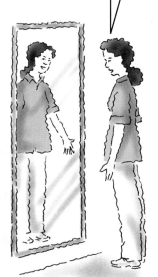

What does a good coworker "look" like? A good coworker impresses others with her consistency, helpfulness, and dedication.

QUESTIONNAIRE TIME!

Are you a good coworker? Take this survey and find out! Just answer the questions by filling in each blank with the appropriate number. For example, if you always show up to work on time, then you would put a "5" next to the first question.

1	2	3	4	5
never	*rarely*	*sometimes*	*usually*	*always*

1. I show up to work on time and ready to start my day. _____
2. I listen to my coworkers' suggestions and criticisms. _____
3. I am a team player. _____
4. I try to schedule my personal days and vacations in a way that's fair to my coworkers. _____
5. I offer assistance to coworkers without being asked first. _____
6. I have a positive and optimistic attitude. _____
7. I treat everyone with the same courtesy and respect. _____
8. I am willing to assume new responsibilities and learn new skills. _____
9. I follow office policies and procedures. _____
10. I make an effort to get along with my coworkers. _____

Now, add up your points to see how you rate!

45–50 points = You're a responsible and dependable coworker. Your coworkers enjoy working with you because you have a good work ethic and good habits.

40–45 = You're a good coworker, although you may have some trouble meeting challenges or honing your skills.

35–40 = You're an average coworker, and sometimes you have problems working up to your full potential. Others may see you as inconsistent or pessimistic.

Below 35 = Your work ethic, habits, and attitude need improvement!

Learning Is a Lifelong Process

Having a great job as a medical assistant can fulfill your professional needs, and you will learn a lot of things through experience. But sometimes, there is only so much you can learn in an office setting. When your day-to-day tasks seem to become repetitive, you may find yourself asking, "What else is out there?"

Well, there is good news for you! Medical technology and science are constantly evolving, and medical professionals must adapt to accommodate new and better patient treatment options. Education is the primary tool you can use to improve yourself as a health care professional.

As you learned in Chapter 1, continuing your education is an important part of medical assisting. Typical subjects covered in continuing education courses and seminars include:

- new techniques or medical procedures
- drugs and vaccines
- insurance coding and billing regulations
- technology—software and hardware

In addition to these topics, many medical offices require employees to receive annual education on cardiopulmonary resuscitation (CPR), infection control, OSHA, and fire and electrical safety.

GIVING CREDIT WHERE CREDIT IS DUE

Continuing education units (CEUs) are awarded to medical assistants who've completed educational programs or courses recognized by the AAMA. You can obtain CEUs by doing the following:

- attending approved local and state AAMA meetings and seminars
- completing guided study courses

- reading appropriate journal articles and submitting a posttest for CEU credit

Once you're a certified medical assistant (CMA), you may obtain recertification every five years by either retaking the examination or completing 60 CEUs in a five-year period. (You'll learn more about recertification later in this chapter.)

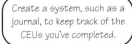

Create a system, such as a journal, to keep track of the CEUs you've completed.

BENEFITS AND CHALLENGES

Like all worthwhile activities, choosing to continue your education can present some unique challenges as well as some surprising benefits. Additional courses and training, outside of those required by your supervisor or office, may be of additional cost to you. However, employers are often willing to pay some of these costs. Also, if you join a professional organization, additional training may be offered at a discount.

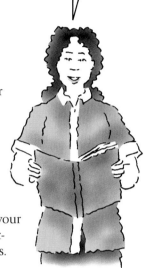

Continuing your education will also take up some of your free time. You may be required to attend events or instructional courses in the evenings, after work, or on weekends. The good news, however, is that many sites offer online courses that can be taken in the comfort of your own home.

OTHER WAYS TO KEEP UP WITH THE TRENDS

Keeping up with trends is about more than remaining "fashionable." Trends in the medical field can mean advances in medical technology, policy and procedural changes, and opportunities for professional growth as a medical assistant. In addition to continuing your education, there are a number of other ways to keep up with the trends in health care and medicine. The following is a list of tips to help you keep up with the latest trends.

- Stay in touch with former instructors, classmates, and peers in the field. Networking keeps you in contact with others who can share new insights and stories with you.

- Watch instructional videos/DVDs. These products can teach you how to adapt a previously learned skill or technique. They also provide information about new procedures or advancements in the field. Speak with your supervisor or the physician regarding where you may obtain these materials.

- Read continuing education articles in professional journals and magazines. If an article is accompanied by a posttest, complete it to gauge how much you've learned.

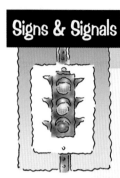

Signs & Signals

FINDING CONTINUING EDUCATION OPPORTUNITIES

You may be thinking that continuing your education sounds like a great idea—if only you knew where to begin. The truth is that educational opportunities are all around you. You need only to know where to look for them! Here are some suggestions to consider when you begin the search for continuing education opportunities:

- Contact the medical assisting program or school from which you graduated. Some schools offer continuing education courses and seminars for graduates.

- Contact former instructors, colleagues, and friends. They may know of opportunities or other people who can help you find continuing education courses.

- Visit the AAMA online at www.aama-ntl.org and apply for membership. As a member, you will be among the first to know about educational opportunities available to you.

Professional Organizations

Networking involves interacting with the people who can help you broaden your career options. One way to network is by joining an appropriate professional organization. But how do you know which organization is right for you?

JOIN UP!

In addition to the opportunity for networking, each organization offers various benefits and incentives for its members. When you join a professional organization, your benefits can include the following:

- access to educational seminars
- access to continuing education units
- subscription to the professional journals that alert you to new procedures and trends in medicine
- access to annual conventions
- group insurance plans

Ask The Professional **WHY SHOULD I JOIN?**

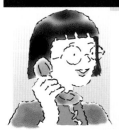

Q: *Why should I join a professional organization if joining is voluntary?*

A: Although joining a professional organization can take some of your time and energy, the benefits you'll receive from joining will make it a worthwhile experience.

Becoming involved in organizations and associations is a great way to network and meet people who can help you find opportunities to continue your education and advance your career. You'll also be among the first to know about medical conferences, events, and opportunities to learn more about medical assisting. Employers are often willing to pay for medical seminars and other educational opportunities. And you can use your new knowledge to improve your skills and expand your career prospects. So what are you waiting for? Choose an organization and sign up today!

You may be interested in signing up but are still wondering, "Where do I begin?" The following are some professional organizations that you might consider. Keep in mind that you can join more than one professional organization.

American Association of Medical Assistants

There are several different levels of membership within the AAMA. But, generally, anyone interested in the medical assisting field may apply for membership. You can apply for membership by visiting the AAMA's website. Once there, either fill out the membership enrollment form online or download and print a hard copy of the form that can be submitted by mail.

Benefits for members include:

- a subscription to *CMA Today*, the AAMA's bimonthly publication, which provides educational articles, current medical news, health policy updates, and association events
- access to the annual AAMA convention with continuing education workshops that offer CEU credits
- discounts available for workshop and seminar fees, self-study courses, and convention registration

- special rates for life insurance and other types of insurance
- opportunities for accreditation, certification, and recertification

American Medical Technologists

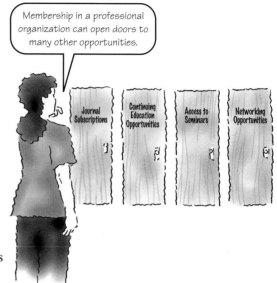

Membership in a professional organization can open doors to many other opportunities.

Members of the AMT include:

- medical technologists
- medical assistants
- dental assistants
- medical laboratory technicians
- office laboratory technicians
- phlebotomy technicians
- laboratory consultants
- allied health instructors
- over 3,000 allied health care students nationwide

Students are eligible to join the AMT for a small fee. Among the benefits for student members are:

- use of the AMT's online job bank, the AMT Career Connection
- eligibility to apply for one of five $500 scholarships (for students pursuing studies in medical laboratory technology, medical assisting, dental assisting, phlebotomy, or office laboratory technician)
- eligibility to take the AMT certification examination

AMT offers certified members a number of additional benefits. Visit their website at www.amt1.com for more information.

American Academy of Professional Coders

The American Academy of Professional Coders (AAPC) offers three types of membership: individual, student, and corporate. If you are no longer a student, then individual membership is the route to take. Visit the organization online at www.aapc.com and click on "Membership" at the top of the page for more information.

Benefits for members include:

- certification opportunities
- specialty-specific credentials
- a subscription to their monthly newsmagazine, *Coding Edge*

- local networking opportunities
- the ability to view job listings and career postings published by the AAPC
- eligibility to attend national and regional conferences
- a subscription to the AAPC's bimonthly e-newsletter, "EDGE BLAST"
- access to professional liability insurance

American Health Information Management Association

The American Health Information Management Association (AHIMA) has different levels of membership as well. Active membership is offered to anyone who is interested in health information management and willing to abide by the organization's code of ethics. Individuals who are currently or were formerly enrolled in an AHIMA-accredited or -approved health information management program are eligible for student membership, which includes the benefits of the AHIMA Mentor Program. If you're interested, visit their website at www.ahima.org to complete an online application or to download and print a hard copy of the application form.

Benefits of membership are many, but some of the highlights include:

- access to Communities of Practice (CoP), a tool for communicating with other members online or by e-mail
- eligibility to attend the AHIMA convention and exhibit
- access to an online library where you can search for journal articles, job descriptions, and AHIMA position statements
- discounts on AHIMA online courses

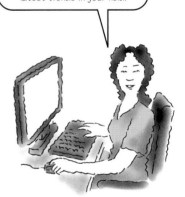

Many professional organizations offer online services. With access to a computer, you can take online courses, chat with other members, and read about the latest trends in your field.

CERTIFICATION AND RENEWAL

As you learned in Chapter 1, graduates of medical assisting programs that are accredited by CAAHEP or ABHES are immediately eligible to take the AAMA's certification examination. Those who pass this test become certified medical assistants (CMAs).

The AMT offers a similar option. Graduates from ABHES-accredited medical assisting programs are immediately eligible to take the registered medical assistant (RMA) examination.

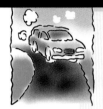

Road Rules — OTHER PROFESSIONAL ORGANIZATIONS

Keep in mind that professional organizations aren't just limited to medical assisting. Depending on the patients you serve and the type of medical practice where you work, you can gain benefits from being in contact with other local and national associations as well, such as:

- professional women's associations
- Alzheimer associations
- diabetes associations
- local support groups

However, graduating from an ABHES- or CAAHEP-accredited medical assisting program is *not* a requirement if the candidate possesses at least five years' experience as a professional medical assistant (spending no more than two of those years as an instructor). Those who meet the necessary requirements can become RMAs.

Becoming a CMA or an RMA improves your education and gives you a title that can help you advance in your career. By becoming certified, you are also eligible to join various associations that promote the medical field and help you meet others interested in medical assisting.

Renewing Your AAMA Certification

A CMA is required to recertify every five years. **Recertification** may be obtained either by taking the examination again or by completing 60 CEUs in a five-year period.

Recertifying by Continuing Education

If you're seeking to recertify your credentials through continuing your education, then your objective is to accumulate 60 recertification points in five years. Thirty of these must be AAMA-approved CEUs. The breakdown of points is as follows:

- 10 administrative
- 10 clinical
- 10 general
- 30 from any combination of the above three categories

Recertification through continued education is a great way to brush up on your skills and knowledge and stay ahead of the trends. It's also a relatively simple process.

1. To make sure that your study time is spent well, you'll need to know which topics will be covered. The AAMA provides three documents that serve as useful guidelines for identifying relevant topics. To access these documents, visit the AAMA's website and click on "Get Recertified" at the top of the page.

2. You have several options for earning recertification points:
   - AAMA self-study courses
   - posttests that follow articles in *CMA Today*
   - continuing education programs and events
   - workshops hosted by local chapters
   - state and local conventions

3. Check your transcript periodically to keep track of the number and types of CEUs you've accumulated. The AAMA keeps a record of your CEUs by adding them to your transcript. (This transcript is similar to your school transcript, which lists all the courses you've taken, the grades you've received, and the credits you've earned.) AAMA members can access their current transcripts online.

It's important to keep your certification up-to-date—and don't forget to update your resume with your new skills, training, and accomplishments!

4. Apply for recertification. You must apply 90 days before your current certification expires. You can download an application form on the AAMA's website.

Recertifying by Examination

If you decide to recertify by examination, you will need to retake the examination for certified medical assistants. You can apply for the test online at the AAMA's website. Once there, highlight "Get Recertified" and select "Recertify by Examination" from the drop-down menu. Then, click on "Apply for the CMA Exam." You can download the application to your computer. To help you prepare for the test, the site offers study resources and the exam outline. Textbook publishers also offer recertification preparation texts. Consider purchasing one if you require additional help.

Continuing Your AMT Certification

The AMT offers a Certification Continuation Program (CCP). Any new member certified on or after January 1, 2006, will be required to provide proof of continuing employment, obtain continuing education every three years, or comply with other ways of meeting CCP criteria.

Depending on your certification, you will be required to obtain a certain number of points over a three-year period. There are several ways to earn points, including:

- earning continuing education credit
- providing an employer evaluation
- authoring published works
- attending instructional presentations

There are no additional fees associated with the CCP program. For more information, visit the AMT's website at www.amt1.com.

The Possibilities Are Endless!

With additional education and training, there are a multitude of positions that become available to you. If you are looking to advance your career in another area, consider the following options.

- *Registered nurse (RN).* Regardless of specialty or work setting, the duties of an RN usually include treating patients, educating patients and the public about various medical conditions, and providing advice and emotional support to patients' family members. RNs record patients' medical histories and symptoms, help perform diagnostic tests and analyze results, operate medical machinery, administer treatment and medications, and help with patient's follow-up and rehabilitation.

- *Registered phlebotomist.* A registered phlebotomist obtains blood specimens by using venipuncture or microtechniques. The phlebotomist aids in the collection and transportation of other laboratory specimens and may also be involved with data entry.

- *Physician assistant (PA).* A PA practices medicine under the supervision of a physician. These professionals perform more advanced skills than medical assistants. PAs are formally trained to provide diagnostic, therapeutic, and preventive health care services as delegated by a physician.

- *Medical assistant instructor.* Most instructors are graduates of a medical assisting programs and have years of experience as medical assistants. Their job is to instruct students learning to be medical assistants.

- *Emergency medical technician (EMT) or paramedic.* With additional training, EMTs and paramedics are able to perform more difficult prehospital medical procedures. These professionals deal with incidents as varied as automobile collisions, heart attacks, drownings, childbirth, and gunshot wounds, all of which require immediate medical attention. EMTs and paramedics provide this vital attention as they care for and transport the sick or injured to medical facilities.

- *Medical office manager.* To become a medical office manager, you must possess a variety of skills and be able to prioritize, juggle responsibilities, and communicate effectively with patients, staff members, and physicians. You must also have strong leadership skills. Managers may be nurses, medical assistants, or administrative support personnel.

CONSIDER YOUR OPTIONS

Seeking new opportunities is essential if your goal is to advance your career. Sometimes, this requires additional training or qualifications. For example, if you're a medical assistant who wishes to become an EMT, you must first complete additional training to learn emergency information and procedures. It's a good idea to research the career you'd like to pursue to learn about any additional costs, training, or licensing required. There is an abundance of available resources online, such as the Department of Labor's website, www.dol.gov. It's also helpful to discuss possible career options with other medical professionals who might be able to provide an "inside look" at the particular field you'd like to pursue.

What career goals do you have in mind? Long-term goals can seem intimidating, but not if they're broken up into smaller, more easily attainable goals over a period of time. Consider what you'd like to be doing in one year. What about five years from now? If it's different from what you're doing now, then consider developing a plan of action to meet your goal.

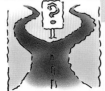

Fork in the Road

WHERE DO YOU WANT TO GO FROM HERE?

Write a short essay (three to five sentences) outlining your career goals for the next five to ten years, including the steps you need to take to reach your goals.

AVOID "JOB-HOPPING"

Sometimes, you find new opportunities that advance your position at your current work site. For example, after you've gained experience and received additional training, your employer may choose to promote you within the office. But at other times, advancing your career may require seeking and applying for a new job altogether.

Each option, whether you choose to stay with your current employer or search for a new job, has its benefits. Working at a new job site can be a great chance to discover what you enjoy doing, meet new people, and expand your resume. However, when you find a job that suits you well, it's best to stick with it. Potential employers like to see that you're a consistent and faithful employee. Frequent job-hopping communicates to potential employers that you have a difficult time committing to a single job or employer. Job-hopping looks bad on your resume and can detract from your other good qualities, such as a strong work ethic and a positive attitude.

> Job-hopping can seem alluring, but too much jumping around can make you appear unreliable to employers. Once you find a job that suits you, stick with it!

Should You Stay or Should You Go?

At one time or another during your career, you'll probably struggle with this question. You may find yourself asking:

- Should I leave this facility where I feel comfortable and safe?
- Will it be worth the transition if I find a job that's better suited to my abilities?
- Would a new job be more financially rewarding?
- Would the benefits be better?

An important factor in many new job searches is salary. However, there are many other considerations to make when deciding whether or not to leave a job. Here are some aspects of a position that are just as important to consider as salary:

- a sense of achievement or of making a personal contribution
- recognition and status

- opportunity for growth and advancement
- harmonious peer relations
- a good working relationship with supervisors
- job security
- comfortable working conditions
- fair company policies
- benefits

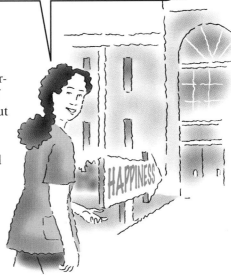

It would be great if you had a sign that could point you in the right direction. But true happiness comes from understanding what you value and using that information to make the decisions that are right for you.

If you're no longer happy at your current position, it may be because one of these elements is missing or lacking. But before you make the decision to leave, ask yourself, "What would make me happier?" Perhaps the supervisor could make a small change to accommodate your needs. For example, if your commute is very time-consuming, adjusting your work hours could solve the problem. Identify the source of your dissatisfaction and propose solutions to your supervisor.

Giving a Proper Good-bye

Choosing whether or not to leave a job can be a tough decision. Changes in life circumstance, geographic location, or changes in family situations are some of the reasons you may choose to leave a job. You may also seek to explore new career options or switch fields. If you do decide to leave your current position, there are several guidelines you should follow to make the transition as smooth as possible for both you and your employer.

- Give adequate notice. A minimum of two weeks' notice is standard, and a month's notice will allow your employer even more time to prepare for your departure and hire a replacement.
- Write a resignation letter explaining why you're leaving. Keep the letter positive. For example, you might write, "I am leaving this position to explore new career opportunities." This letter is usually the last item in your personnel file, so be courteous and respectful of the job and your employer.

- Be positive in your exit interview. Avoid making angry statements about the office or other employees.
- Offer suggestions and constructive criticism for the future.
- Clean and empty your desk, locker, and any other personal space that you used.
- Return any equipment that has been assigned to you.
- Finish all duties and tie up any loose ends. Let your supervisor know about any unfinished business.
- Request a letter of reference.

Following the guidelines above are also important if you'd like a recommendation for another job or might seek to be rehired in the future.

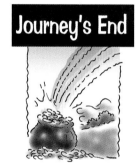

Journey's End

- Having sound technical and soft skills will help you communicate effectively with patients and provide quality care and treatment.
- Abiding by the medical assisting standards of ethics and conduct includes handling mistakes properly, maintaining professional boundaries, and working within your scope of practice.
- Taking initiative, assuming new responsibilities, and finding a mentor are three ways you can show interest in your job and employer.
- Building good rapport with experienced coworkers will help you find a mentor who can provide guidance as you begin your new career.
- Being a respectful and dependable coworker is achieved by showing your support for others, helping where and when you can, and being a team player.
- Continuing your education and keeping up with the trends in health care will help you improve your skills as a medical assistant and expand your career opportunities.
- Renewing your certification and joining a professional organization will allow you to network with others who can provide you with career options for the future.
- Determining your career goals and developing a plan for achieving them are essential to a successful career.
- When considering leaving a job, it's important to examine your level of professional fulfillment, as well as the benefits and challenges of moving on.

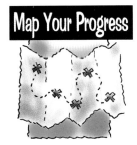

Answer the following multiple-choice questions.

1. What is *impartiality?*
   a. the ability to treat all patients equally, with the same care and concern
   b. the art of handling people with genuine concern and sensitivity
   c. the ability to understand how someone is feeling
   d. the ability to provide a dependable service

2. What does the AAMA Medical Assistant Creed contain?
   a. information about the latest trends in medical technology
   b. a list of common medical office policies and procedures
   c. the principles of the medical assisting profession
   d. a list of tasks commonly performed by medical assistants

3. Why should you avoid working outside your *scope of practice?*
   a. because it is rude to assume the job of a physician
   b. because you don't have the skills or training to perform tasks outside your scope of practice
   c. because your scope of practice is large enough to complete every task available to you
   d. because your scope of practice lets others know what you're trained to do

4. Why should you always report your mistakes to your supervisor?
   a. because your supervisor must dock your pay
   b. because doing so may prevent further harm or legal complications
   c. because your supervisor will need to cover up any mistakes you make
   d. because doing so lets patients know that you're not perfect

5. Adhering to boundaries means that your interactions with patients must always remain:
   a. secretive.
   b. professional.
   c. impersonal.
   d. anonymous.

6. What is an *incident report?*
   a. an article describing working conditions in the office
   b. a series of written statements from patients regarding the quality of their visits
   c. a written account of any negative patient, visitor, or staff event
   d. a document that tracks the number of patients' visits to the office

7. What is the primary way in which you can show interest in your job and employer?
   a. obtaining credentials
   b. showing initiative
   c. giving advice
   d. being punctual

8. Which of the following is *not* one of the benefits of joining a professional organization?
   a. networking
   b. career advancement opportunities
   c. continuing education opportunities
   d. increased vacation time

9. A registered phlebotomist:
   a. takes patients' vital signs.
   b. transports patients to the hospital during emergencies.
   c. instructs medical assisting students.
   d. obtains patients' blood specimens.

10. Why is job-hopping a bad idea?
    a. because employers want to see that you're a consistent and dependable worker
    b. because it's expensive to change jobs
    c. because your current supervisor and coworkers are counting on you
    d. because the patients have become comfortable with you

GLOSSARY

accreditation A nongovernmental professional peer review process that provides technical assistance and evaluates educational programs for quality based on preestablished academic and administrative standards [Chapter 1]

Accrediting Bureau of Health Education Schools (ABHES) A professional organization that identifies specific skills and information that accredited medical assisting programs must teach students [Chapter 1]

active listening Being mentally and physically engaged with what the other person is saying; listening for meaning [Chapter 2]

American Association of Medical Assistants (AAMA) Professional organization for medical assistants [Chapter 1]

American Medical Technologists (AMT) Professional organization for medical assistants, medical laboratory technicians, dental assistants, and other allied health students and professionals [Chapter 1]

anacusis Complete hearing loss [Chapter 4]

attitude A state of mind; how a person feels about a given subject or at a given time [Chapter 1]

autism A developmental disability that affects communication, social interaction, and creative or imaginative play; the disorder is usually identified during early childhood and persists throughout adulthood [Chapter 4]

bias Formation of an opinion without foundation or reason; prejudice [Chapter 4]

bilingual Able to speak and understand two languages [Chapter 4]

cerebral palsy A developmental disability caused by damage to the cerebrum, the part of the brain involved with motor control [Chapter 4]

certification Voluntary process that involves a testing procedure to prove an individual's competency in a particular area [Chapter 1]

chain of infection The six key conditions that must be met for a person to contract a communicable infection (pathogen, reservoir, portal of exit, method of transmission, portal of entry, and susceptible host) [Chapter 4]

clarification Explanation; removal of confusion or uncertainty [Chapter 2]

clinical coordinator Medical administrative professional who matches students to appropriate externship sites chosen by the school [Chapter 5]

Commission on Accreditation of Allied Health Education Programs (CAAHEP) A professional organization that identifies specific skills that accredited medical assisting programs must teach students [Chapter 1]

communicable infections Infections that can be spread from one person to another [Chapter 4]

congenital Adjective that is used to describe a disorder that a person is born with [Chapter 4]

contaminated Polluted; possessing infectious organisms or substances [Chapter 4]

continuing education Courses and seminars on various topics of education that occur after a student has completed her medical assisting program [Chapter 1]

continuing education units (CEUs) Credits awarded for attendance at approved local and state AAMA meetings and seminars, completion of guided study courses, and journal articles designed to submit a posttest for CEU credit [Chapter 7]

courtesy Politeness; respectfulness [Chapter 2]

cultural diversity The differences that individuals and groups bring to a culture; ethnic, gender, racial, and socioeconomic variety in a situation, institution, or group [Chapter 4]

culture The shared beliefs, customs, and attitudes that provide social structure for daily living [Chapter 4]

customer service Refers to the ways you help customers have a positive experience [Chapter 3]

dementia Progressive and permanent loss of the ability to think and remember, caused by damage to the brain tissue [Chapter 4]

developmental disabilities Permanent disabilities that affect people before they reach adulthood and interfere with their abilities to reach developmental milestones [Chapter 4]

diplomacy The art of handling people with tact and genuine concern [Chapter 3]

discrimination The act of making a difference in favor of or against someone [Chapter 4]

Down syndrome A developmental disability that is the result of having an extra chromosome; people with this disorder have mental retardation and certain key physical features, such as almond-shaped eyes and short stature [Chapter 4]

dysphagia Inability to swallow or difficulty in swallowing [Chapter 4]

empathy The ability to understand or to some extent share what someone else is feeling [Chapter 2]

ethics Guidelines for moral behavior that are enforced by peer groups [Chapter 1]

ethnocentrism The belief that one's own ideas, beliefs, and practices are superior and preferable to others [Chapter 4]

externship An educational course that allows the student to obtain hands-on experience [Chapters 1, 5]

feedback In communication, the response to input from another person [Chapter 2]

Health Insurance Portability and Accountability Act (HIPAA) Federal law that requires all health care settings to ensure privacy and security of patient information [Chapter 1]

incident report A written account of any negative patient, visitor, or staff event [Chapter 7]

infection control Basic practices designed to decrease the chance that an infection will spread from one person to another in a health care facility [Chapter 4]

integrity Honesty; when what you say and what you do are one and the same [Chapter 1]

kinesics A form of nonverbal communication including facial expressions, gestures, and body movements [Chapter 2]

medical ethics Principles that govern the behavior and conduct of health professionals in terms of proper medical etiquette, customs, and professional courtesy [Chapter 1]

mentor Person who shares experience, knowledge, and wisdom about a particular occupation or about the workplace in general [Chapter 5]

multiple sclerosis (MS) Disorder that affects the nervous system, typically causing muscle weakness and eventual paralysis [Chapter 4]

muscular dystrophy An inherited disease that causes the skeletal muscles to become weaker over time [Chapter 4]

networking A system of personal and professional relationships through which to share information [Chapter 6]

nonlanguage Not expressed in spoken language, e.g., laughing, sobbing, grunting, sighing [Chapter 2]

paralanguage Factors connected with, but not essentially part of language, e.g., tone of voice, volume, pitch [Chapter 2]

paralysis Impaired movement or a complete loss of voluntary muscle movement in certain parts of the body [Chapter 4]

paraphrasing Restating what you hear using your own words [Chapter 2]

personal protective equipment (PPE) Equipment such as disposable gloves, gowns, masks, and protective eyewear that protects a person from exposure to blood or other body fluids [Chapter 4]

portfolio A portable case containing documents [Chapter 6]

preceptor Graduate medical assistant, licensed practical nurse, or registered nurse who instructs medical assisting students at an externship site [Chapter 5]

professionalism The attitude of being a professional; having a positive outlook and a commitment to doing your best at work at all times; the ability to use your knowledge and skills to secure the interests and welfare of patients [Chapter 1]

proxemics Having to do with the physical space between two people who are communicating [Chapter 2]

rapport Mutual feelings of trust and respect shared between people in a healthy relationship [Chapter 1]

recertification Certification renewed either by taking the examination again or by completing a specified number of continuing education units in a five-year period [Chapter 7]

reflecting Repeating what you hear using open-ended phrases or questions [Chapter 2]

scope of practice The range of tasks you're allowed to perform due to the level of your training or abilities [Chapter 7]

service animal Any animal that has been trained to provide assistance to a person with a disability [Chapter 4]

special needs Medical conditions that require special care and consideration from medical staff, family members, and others [Chapter 4]

stereotyping Holding an opinion of all members of a particular culture or group based on oversimplified or negative characterizations [Chapter 4]

summarizing Reviewing briefly what the patient tells you [Chapter 2]

INDEX